T0171378

I GAVE MYSELF CANCER,

I CAN TAKE IT AWAY!

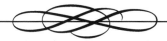

ALTERNATIVES BROUGHT ME BACK TO LIFE.

Linda Christina Beauregard

BALBOA.
PRESS
A DIVISION OF HAY HOUSE

Balboa Press books may be ordered through booksellers or by contacting:

Balboa Press
A Division of Hay House
1663 Liberty Drive
Bloomington, IN 47403
www.balboapress.com
1-(877) 407-4847

Because of the dynamic nature of the Internet, any web addresses or links contained in this book may have changed since publication and may no longer be valid. The views expressed in this work are solely those of the author and do not necessarily reflect the views of the publisher, and the publisher hereby disclaims any responsibility for them.

The author of this book does not dispense medical advice or prescribe the use of any technique as a form of treatment for physical, emotional, or medical problems without the advice of a physician, either directly or indirectly. The intent of the author is only to offer information of a general nature to help you in your quest for emotional and spiritual well-being. In the event you use any of the information in this book for yourself, which is your constitutional right, the author and the publisher assume no responsibility for your actions.

Any people depicted in stock imagery provided by Thinkstock are models, and such images are being used for illustrative purposes only. Certain stock imagery © Thinkstock.

Printed in the United States of America.

ISBN: 978-1-4525-7136-2 (sc)
ISBN: 978-1-4525-7137-9 (hc)
ISBN: 978-1-4525-7138-6 (e)

Library of Congress Control Number: 2013905545

Balboa Press rev. date: 4/24/2013

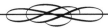

THIS BOOK IS DEDICATED TO my late father, Paul R. Beauregard, who I never really knew or understood until very recently. His love came pouring through to me in a recent evidential-medium reading I experienced.

As you said to me, Dad, "You have a bit of a responsibility, girl, to make up for me."

You were also right about my transparency, Dad. Yes, I am transparent, from the heart. Thank you for coming back to me and showing me what I needed to do—complete this story and share it with the world.

This is a tribute to a cherished father I never knew and who I long to embrace and love for the first time.

CONTENTS

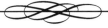

DISCLAIMER

THIS BOOK IS FOR INFORMATIONAL purposes only and is not intended as medical advice, as a substitute for medical counseling, or as a treatment or cure for any disease or health condition and should not be construed as such. It is not intended as a substitute for the diagnosis, treatment, or advice from a qualified, licensed professional. Always work with a qualified health professional before making any changes to your lifestyle, diet, and prescription drug use or exercise activities. No one should consider that this book represents the practice of medicine. This book assumes no responsibility for how the material herein is used. Please be advised that the statements regarding alternative treatments for cancer have not been evaluated by the FDA.

While I make repeated references to various name brand products and supplements I do not specifically endorse any of them or have any association with the product or supplement manufacturers.

PREFACE

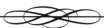

THE PURPOSE OF THIS BOOK is to create an awareness of alternative methods of caring for your body and your health. This isn't another diet or recipe book. It's a lifestyle book focused on how the choices you make on a daily basis can turn your health around in a flash, in the blink of an eye. You don't have to use only the methods offered by the mainstream medical community when and if you get sick. There are many alternative options available to choose from, more than those I will mention here.

In this book, I will share with you a very personal, intimate, sometimes humorous, and detailed story of my own return to health using only alternative options after an initial lumpectomy that brought a diagnosis of breast cancer. Unfortunately, most, if not all, of these alternatives are not available from the menu of options offered by conventional medicine.

So here I am, passion overflowing and blessed with this incredible opportunity to spread the word about alternative treatment options. You do have choices. There are many alternative healing methods available should you find yourself in a compromised state of health and looking for information outside of mainstream medicine. You just have to do your research on the Internet, talk to family and friends, talk to organic farmers, go to the bookstore, and look into natural healing magazines to find out what they are, where they're offered, and how you can benefit from them.

All kinds of cancer and other diseases are rampant in our country; we all know this. All you need to do is listen to the news or your friends or pick up a paper or magazine. People compare notes on which doctor to use for what. Is their bedside manner soft or harsh? Do they make things easy to understand or difficult? Are they a success in their community? You hear it almost every minute of every day, if you're inclined to be in those circles.

After being diagnosed with breast cancer in 2005, I chose a most unusual path to my recovery. I chose to use alternative solutions exclusively, solutions not considered viable options by mainstream medicine. I cured—yes, *cured*—my breast cancer without using additional surgery, chemotherapy, radiation, or other drugs.

I thought that fighting this disease was going to be the biggest battle of my life. It turned out the greatest challenge was to obtain information from the medical community about the power of alternative solutions. Alternatives are incredibly powerful, but the medical community doesn't readily recognize the force and the power of proper food, physical detoxification, vitamin and mineral supplementation, and spiritual practices as possible solutions to reverse disease.

I Gave Myself Cancer, I Can Take It Away is my testimonial about my journey and how I overcame breast cancer with these alternatives. Most of my family and friends thought I was crazy, and at times I thought so too. It was a lonely journey, and I had almost no one to turn to or talk with about the direction I chose. There were no *alternative* support groups available to share experiences. No one believed in me except my sister Patti and the people who were counseling me at HealthQuarters in Colorado Springs, Colorado.

I'm here because what I discovered along the path of this journey was profoundly intense yet so simple and easy that even I couldn't believe that I cured myself of cancer in just five months. What I discovered was the power of plants (POP) and organic, raw, living fruits and vegetables, as well as the power of believing in myself and my connection to a higher source. I followed my intuition. As it turned out, once given the tools it needed, my body healed from what is typically recognized as a deadly disease—breast cancer. I not only healed myself of the cancer, but I lost thirty pounds, felt fabulous, and looked great!

After more than seven years on this new diet and some lifestyle changes, I can tell you life is far better than ever before cancer. Since employing all the means I'll identify in the following pages, I don't take any prescription drugs, and I don't use over-the-counter medications even for a rare headache.

You can be incredibly healthy, live vibrantly, and live long.

You just have to want it, believe you can have it, and practice it. I plan to live at least to 115, and I won't experience any disease along the way. No, I'm not neurotic or a purist about my new lifestyle. I still enjoy an occasional cocktail and I don't fret about eating a non-organic meal if I'm dining out, but these are infrequent departures from what I've learned to love. So you don't need to give up living to have a life. It's not a trade-off, it's a compromise—a beautiful, life-giving, life-sustaining compromise.

Why do I say, feel, and predict the things I do regarding my health? I've lived them and intend to keep on living them, and I want to share my personal breast-cancer recovery story and how my decisions have impacted me, my family, and friends.

My successful recovery from breast cancer without conventional and traditional methods like additional surgery, chemotherapy, radiation, and drug therapy (otherwise known as cutting, burning, and poisoning) has been labeled anecdotal. I don't need anyone's opinion about what happened to me because I was the one who lived through my recovery. I know exactly how and why I got sick and what I did to get well. I want you to be the recipient of my experience, because these practices worked for me, and they may work for you, too.

You don't have to succumb to the diagnosis, no matter what it is. Your age, gender, or predispositions to family history of genetic medical conditions or diseases thought to be *hereditary* are, for the most part, irrelevant. You have been conditioned by the diet and lifestyle you currently live. You can change that. You can overcome just about any illness, including cancer, diabetes, heart disease, osteoporosis, and arthritis—among many others—without harmful side effects. The last chapter in this book contains some very convincing testimonials from people who completely recovered from life threatening diseases and death sentences using alternative solutions. Some of these people actually tried conventional treatments first, that failed. Imagine that.

I hope you're reading this book because you want to improve your health and your life and not because you're already in a state of disrepair. But if your body is in need of serious help, have no fear. Whatever your diagnosis, it's not a death sentence. I hope you become inspired to take a closer look at your diet, exercise, and mental and spiritual approach to life. These are all key elements in any recovery plan and will turn your health and your life around.

You no longer need to be a victim. Embrace your God-given right to make your own choices and decisions. Melt away mediocre thinking and wake up to the wonder of you. Be larger than life, because you are. You just need someone to convince you that you can. Expand your beliefs, and awaken your heart. Vibrant health and radiant living are right around the corner. They are your birthright.

Read on, take charge of your own health, and place the overall responsibility back where it belongs: in your most capable hands. Don't look any further; you have the power; you are in charge. I did it. Thousands of others have done it, and so can you!

ACKNOWLEDGMENTS

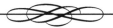

THANKS TO DR. DAVID AND his wife Anne Frahm, founders of HealthQuarters Ministries in Colorado Springs, and to all their staff engaged in the co-creation of rebuilding life. Their spoken and written words about surviving cancer and other diseases gave me the courage to think about the incredible healing nature of my own body. HealthQuarters further inspired me to engage a path of learning that would ultimately change my life and the lives of many of my family and friends.

My deep gratitude and appreciation to my sister Patricia Dwyer for all the support and comfort she gave me when no one else would. I was certainly thinking outside the box and outside of the offerings of mainstream medicine. Thanks for coming to HealthQuarters Ministries in Colorado Springs with me, for all the prayers you offered, the confidence you placed in my choice of treatments, and for investing emotionally in my recovery. We found out together that we could live without morning coffee and stuffing our faces full of carbohydrates and nighttime cocktails! You were my reinforcement when I was down, and you stood by my side through all the laughter, tears, and early-morning phone calls as we discussed my morning enema results, juicing, raw food recipes, and which vitamins and supplements to take. It was all worth it! I love you.

How to express something words almost cannot? Thanks to one of the best friends anyone could have, a guide and a supporter who continued to encourage me to write this book at times when I felt ill-equipped to do so. He saw qualities and a depth in me I never knew existed, and I admire and love him for the comforting words he shared with me to cheer me on and to become more. I did become more, and he will always have a place in my heart. Thank you, Barry Fuss, for all the wonderful spiritual and emotional gifts you gave me.

Thanks to Frederic Delarue, French author and musical composer, for the clarity I received in moving forward to share my story from reading his book, *Eyes of Your Heart*. The angelic sound waves of his music warmly caress my heart and soothe every cell in my body. I relax into the love and light of my own connection to source energy, my God. (Delarue 2009)

Thank you to yet another great friend, Nancy Condit-Fitzgerald, who continues to stand by me after more than thirty years of wonderful friendship. I will love you forever.

INTRODUCTION

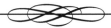

YOU HAVE VALUE—GREATER VALUE THAN you know. You are powerful— more powerful than you know. You are loved— more loved than you know. You have choices.

Whoa! Put the brakes on! You have choices? Where are the choices in our health-care system?

Yes, you do have choices, but only if you're informed about what they are and where to find them. You probably won't find your regular medical doctor suggesting some of them because these choices don't involve toxic drugs, surgery, and radiation or chemotherapy cocktails. You won't find these options lurking in a pill or a potion from your doctor or hospital. You have to dig a little deeper, beyond traditional means.

I was fifty years old when I was diagnosed with breast cancer. I wasn't a bit happy about the possibility of dying at an earlier age than my mother who died at fifty seven from lung cancer. She was a three-pack-a-day smoker all her adult life, and my father smoked just as much as she did. For some reason I was able to escape completely the desire or need to engage in that dirty and addictive habit. My exposure to smoking was second hand with the exception of a very short-lived experimentation during high school.

Smoke filled our house even before breakfast. I grew up seeing my mother and father wake up in the morning, already short-winded and coughing, looking for their fist cigarette of the day. At the breakfast table—just me and my parents—the smoke filled the air like a late-night bar scene. So that was it; I was not going to follow in my parents' smoky footsteps. My memory of this is like it was yesterday: my parents holding a cigarette in between their index and middle fingers first thing in the morning, coughing and hacking while taking a puff and blowing it out one side of their mouths while trying to communicate out of the other. Somewhere in between puffs they found a way to eat their Standard American Diet (SAD) breakfast of fried eggs, bacon, buttered toast, and coffee.

They were addicted to a horrible, major, life-altering—not to mention life-threatening— habit. From this, I learned a lesson so well that growing up in the sixties' and seventies' I could never bring myself to try smoking a marijuana cigarette or experiment with any other so-called recreational drugs. Smoking possibilities of any kind were off the radar. Thanks mom and dad; that was a good thing. I certainly had plenty of opportunity to try drugs, but I wasn't interested. My friends frequently dabbled in many of the popular recreational drugs available at the time. I guess that's why I was a bit isolated from them, but that's a story for another time.

Through my search for cancer cures I discovered that all disease is a condition of an immune system malfunction and a starving body, a body that could be eating plenty but hungry for the right kinds of nutrients. We eat dead food. Yes, we eat food that's been way over-processed. We eat refined food to which fillers of unknown origin have been added and nutrients washed away. We eat over-heated, bottled, frozen, imitation, boxed-up excuses for food.

Until we get back to the garden and start consuming more fresh organic fruits, vegetables, and juices, which are loaded with living enzymes and dense with Mother Earth's version of vitamins and minerals, we're going to continue to be sick and get sicker. One recent evening news report I heard shared information about the increasing number of allergies in very young people. It's really no surprise; they've been fed a diet of dead food their entire lives. How can a body function on dead food? It just can't, and I know this now. Enzymes are part of the solution, and we'll learn more about them later.

Up until I was diagnosed, I thought I was eating a healthy diet. I watched all the ads on TV, and thought: *TV is like God, isn't it?*

I grew up on the old food pyramid that was the source of our diet in the fifties and sixties. Meat was at the bottom: you needed three servings a day. Then came grains, vegetables, fruits, and everything else in moderation on top. I was convinced these things weren't bad for me, and the marketing for these products made them seem so right. My mother prepared what she thought were healthy meals. We had plenty of red meat, white meat, and even pork—the other white meat—, potatoes, and some kind of vegetable at every meal, all cooked. Dessert was only available if either of us had time to bake, or sometimes she bought a Freihofer's Pecan Coffee Ring, one of her other favorite store-bought desserts.

I must say all of those foods were good-tasting, but were they life-sustaining? What did I know? It was all I ever experienced. Like mother, like daughter. We had dead meat smothered in gravy and dead vegetables smothered in butter and salt and pepper. Oh, I almost forgot, cheese and diet soda were two other staples of my diet. In my later years, Bill, my former husband, and I could eat eight ounces of cheese and half a box of crackers before dinner and then sit down and eat a regular meal on top of that, just like I had growing up.

Our parents only pass down from one generation to the next what they learned or were taught from their parents. Is it any wonder *family history* generates *family expected* diseases? We eat the same bad diets and probably assume the same bad health and lifestyle patterns our parents, grandparents, and great grandparents did. Our makeup is one of family history. Voila! You're going to get what your ancestors got. So if you want to live like you've never lived before, change your diet and change your life.

As I grew up, moved out of the house, and began a career, I started to meet people whose diets I wouldn't dare even consider: *vegetarians*. What were they thinking? Meat was a necessity of life. If we didn't eat meat we would surely die, and what kind of person didn't eat meat anyway? Vegetarians were a little scary, and what planet did these aliens come from?

There was even a young man I worked with who did a *fast*. What was that all about? Well, I was soon to find out.

My mother's side of the family had longevity. Had it not been for the smoking, I'm sure she would have lived a much longer life. My grandmother and aunt on my mother's side of the family both lived to be ninety three. My Aunt Jeannette is still alive as the only remaining member of the nineteen siblings on my mom's side, and she's eighty eight. She still mows her own lawn and shovels her own sidewalk in the winter. She's an incredible woman.

My grandparents lived on a farm and raised their own food, from meat and poultry to fresh fruits and vegetables. Many people say that their parents and grandparents ate meat and lived to be close to one-hundred years of age and that they don't understand why meat and dairy products are no longer healthy for you. Here are three reasons why. *Pesticides* are used to grow food that animals are given to eat. *Hormones* are given to the animals to quickly fatten them so they yield more pounds per animal, thereby yielding more profit per animal for the commercial farmer. And last are the *antibiotics* administered to control the health of animals that are forced to live and grow in the most deplorable conditions.

I recently had the misfortune of witnessing first-hand the living conditions that these animals are forced to endure. Yes, you see it presented in documentaries and you see it on the news, but nothing can prepare you for the actual experience of a first-hand viewing of confined animals standing in wretched and miserable conditions and constricted from moving and grazing about freely, just waiting to be fattened up and slaughtered. The smell of the farm was even more reprehensible. Where's the fresh air for these animals and the people who work on these farms?

None of these chemically-based additives were given to animals in our grandparents' time, and consequently none of these chemicals were found in the meat or meat by-products (milk, cheese, yogurt, eggs, etc.). If our grandparents had dairy cows, they used the milk fresh from the cow. It didn't go through any pasteurization or homogenization process. After a lifetime of consuming chemically poisoned meat, meat by-products, and dead dairy products is it any wonder people get cancer and all kinds of other diseases as well? I think not.

The same is true for our produce. Chemical fertilizers and pesticides are put into the soil and sprayed onto the fruits and vegetables to enhance the size and look of every apple and cantaloupe and every tomato, green pepper, and head of broccoli and lettuce farmed in this way. Again, more chemical soup goes on food we know is *supposed* to nourish us. No one questions the need for and the importance of fresh fruits and vegetables in our diet. But what happens to these chemicals once they're sprayed onto the crops and the soil around the crops? After the crops absorb what they can, the runoff goes into the soil and eventually ends up in our water supply, polluting our fresh drinking water, streams, and lakes and eventually the oceans. The toxic load the fish and animals take on as a result of this pollution in the air and water supply creates a domino effect and a vicious cycle of contamination.

Our grandparents of the late nineteenth century did not use chemicals to grow their food, so consuming smaller fruits and vegetables with a little blemish here or there was acceptable. They just cut off the blemish and moved on. Why do we need *perfect*-looking produce anyway? What's wrong with a little blemish here or there as long as Mother Nature put it there? I would rather have smaller produce with a little blemish than know I'm consuming a plateful of mysterious toxic chemicals, the origins of which are unknown. Again, here is the marketing industry, in the interest of big business, telling us that anything but perfect-looking food is not acceptable. The competition to have good-looking food is in the financial interest of big business and not in the best interest of our health.

We've become living, breathing experiments. But we don't have to become test subjects in any experiment as long as we take responsibility for our health and use our common sense to decipher all the marketing out there that's used to help big industry get bigger. The point is *we must* accept and become responsible for our own health if we are going to live long, healthy, productive lives.

The only answer is to eat organically-grown produce and free-range meat from animals fed with organically grown feed or naturally grass-fed if the animals are the grazing kind. That is, if you even want to eat meat after reading the other reasons for not doing so that I will get into later.

Over the last sixty plus years, the food pyramid has been influenced by the amount of money poured into lobbying politicians by various meat, dairy, sugar, or other food *manufacturing* industries. Dr. T. Colin Campbell, a well respected health advocate and author of *The China Study: Startling Implications for Diet, Weight Loss and Long-term Health*, discusses the food pyramid in an article called "The Food Pyramid" and he tells it like it is. As a participating member of several diet and health panels in the past he has some insight to share that suggests our government representatives are more interested in power, money and position than our health. (ezHealthyDiet.com 2007).

Just as an example, the total amount of overall lobbying spending rose from $1.44 billion in 1998 to $3.3 billion at the end of 2012. (OpenSecrets.org "Lobbying Database" 2013) In 2012, reporting by Agribusiness showed the top two sub-lobbying groups to be the Agricultural Services/Products and Food Processing and Sales. Their spending on lobbying for 2012 alone was $33,715,874 and $28,912,686 respectively. (OpenSecrets.org "Agribusiness" 2013) Monsanto was the top spender, contributing $5,970,000, and the American Farm Bureau contributed $5,694,421 in the Agricultural Services/ Products division. (OpenSecrets.org "Agricultural Services/Products" 2013) Nestle SA and the Grocery Manufacturers Association contributed $3,571,645 and $3,350,000 respectively in the Food Processing Sales division. (OenSecrets.org "Food Processing & Sales" 2013) Familiar names like the CropLife America, Kraft Foods Group, Kellogg Co., General Mills and Tyson Foods were close behind along with chemical and fertilizer companies. Just imagine how much influence can be bought with those millions of dollars and how much good could actually be accomplished if that money was spent on supporting organic sustainable farming instead of lobbying. (OpenSecrets. org 2013)

The air and water we breathe and drink are polluted with all kinds of minute toxic chemicals that are approved by the authorities who are supposed to protect us, but for the most part act in the interest of big business. How much of a bad thing, even as it's taken in small doses, does it take, over time, to offset our body's immune system and generate illness? Toxic overload is the result, and our body revolts in the form of disease.

Who are they really protecting? It's big industry that pollutes our water and air with their dumping, commercial farming, and toxic manufacturing by-products. Add to this formula the choice of a stressful lifestyle, and you're guaranteed to get some kind of serious health malfunction, disease, or cancer.

The term "farm to table" has gone by the wayside. Now we look to manufacturing to bring processed food to our tables. Is that what we want, or more importantly, what we need? The information I uncovered as I dove into reading book upon book and article upon article about what foods and additives may cause cancer and other diseases left me feeling like I had been scammed into thinking the diet I consumed for fifty years was actually good for me.

"Let food be thy medicine and medicine be thy food." Hippocrates said that in 400 BCE. We've come so far away from this that it's reprehensible how mainstream medicine uses all kinds of toxic, potent, harmful, and life-threatening drugs in the name of healthy treatments and prospective cures. Because of the quantity of pharmaceutical drugs being prescribed and taken, many people experience side effects that are in and of themselves debilitating and sometimes worse than the condition being treated. More than half of the adult population, ranging in age between fifty seven and eighty five, are taking at least five or more prescription drugs a day. This frequently creates a vast complex of interactions, some of which may include possible death. (Natural News.com "Baby boomers - Why detoxifying toxins from your early years could save your life" 2013)

When you see commercials for prescription drugs on television, how do you feel? I hear the narrator asking if you're experiencing one or more various symptoms for a drug they're marketing. I see the actor in a great state of discomfort before taking the drug and then suddenly behaving euphoric, smiling, romping around and loving life again; apparently the problem is solved. All that takes about ten seconds. Then it starts. The longest portion of time devoted to the commercial is for the disclaimer and side effect warnings: the long and extensive list of side effects. Vomiting, diarrhea, headache, do not combine with this drug or that drug, do not take if this condition or another condition is present, do not take if pregnant, etc. This all ends with "Ask your doctor." And I'm sure the doctor has a plentiful supply of samples to dole out, too.

Do you want to take these drugs, feel like you're already dead, and then live another ten years before you actually die? Do you want to treat one health problem with a drug that may cause several other health challenges? Or do you want to live a vibrant, active, and truly healthy life right now, right up to the end? Organic fruits and vegetables in the produce department seem very friendly now, don't they?

You have complete control over most cancer-causing elements you use and consume in your home such as the food you choose to eat, the water you drink, the air you breathe, the laundry products you use, and the cosmetics, lotions, and colognes you put on your face and body. Others, like the food, air, and water you consume outside of your home, you have much less control over. However, when our government, which we thought was there to protect us, appears to be primarily protecting the profits of special interest corporations, especially the chemical and pharmaceutical industries, then you're left with the one thing you can control, *you*, and the choices you make every day in your life. Your choices will make a difference, a *huge* difference. I'm living proof of this, as are so many other people like me.

I would like you to understand just how easy it is to regain your health once you've lost it and maintain a state of well-being quite unimaginable by today's standards. By using primarily what's in the produce section of your neighborhood grocery store, your local farmers market, and local food cooperatives, you will get well and stay that way. Four other important pieces to your recovery plan include: ridding your body of deadly toxic chemicals, taking vitamin and mineral supplements to rebuild your immune system, eliminating fear from your life, and connecting with a belief system that really works for you and not against you.

Toxic chemicals are not part of the body's makeup, and what does a body do with all the ingested chemicals? Over time and with a weakened immune system the body starts to show symptoms of disease, and cancer is just one of them. And the medical community, the big pharmaceutical companies, and well-intentioned businesses are in a spin trying to raise money to find a cure for this or that kind of cancer or other diseases. It sickens me to see how much money is contributed to non-profit charitable organizations like the American Cancer Society, the American Lung Association or the American Heart Association, the American Diabetes Association and many others, all fighting against something and looking for cures. The cures are already here. The answers lie in the quality of our food choices, diets and lifestyles. It is really that simple. Again, imagine all that money being spent to support life-sustaining organic farming. Oh Joy!

Part of the problem as I see it is that alternative options are not readily available through mainstream medicine, so doctors don't tell you about them. And when you bring a suggestion to your doctor like *juicing*, you get the *stupid* look—the "You have to be kidding me" look. That's way too simple to work. Juicing versus chemotherapy? In my opinion, juicing will win hands down every time. Your doctor may say you need hard-core toxic chemical chemotherapy cocktails to knock out your cancer along with radiation and perhaps surgery. Raw fruits and vegetables, raw juices, wheatgrass juice, green smoothies, vitamin supplements, detoxing, visualization—no, that's too easy. I've been there, done that, and I'm here to share with you that *yes*, it is that easy; these things do work! Alternatives, especially organic fruits and vegetables, are more powerful than toxic drugs, and there are *no* harmful side effects.

While I make repeated references to my dissatisfaction with the medical community regarding their solutions and treatments for illness and disease, I mean no disrespect to their dedication to helping people. The medical community is sometimes guided by forces outside itself—namely the pharmaceutical industry, government agencies, and big business. I would certainly not deny treatment in the event of a medical emergency due to an accident. Traditional medicine has a place, a very valuable place, in diagnostics and emergency medicine among others. Yet when it comes to treatments for disease, there are better, much better options.

You no longer need to be a victim. Embrace your God-given right to make your own decisions. Melt away mediocre thinking and wake up to the wonder of you. Be larger than life, because you are, you just need someone to show you how. Let fear fall by the wayside, expand your beliefs, and awaken your heart. Vibrant health and radiant living are your birthright. Go get them!

CHAPTER 1

Do You Want to Live or
Do You Want to Die?

D O YOU WANT TO LIVE, or do you want to die? You may think that's a really crazy question. Doesn't everyone want to live? How you live and how healthy you are while here on this earth are the real issues. Everyone is going to die at some point, right? But how you go down at the end can be a direct result of the choices you make along the way. Many elderly people who live in nursing homes that are more like halfway houses on their way to knocking on death's door may really want to die; they are ready to embrace death and are eager for its arrival.

They are burdened with Alzheimer's and other diseases; they don't recognize their family or friends anymore and are wasting away both physically and mentally.

Have they given up on life? Have they decided now is their time to die? Could the consequences of their choices have put them in this compromised state of health much earlier than if a different set of choices had been made? Could they have made better diet and lifestyle choices that would have extended their lives and made them vibrant, fit, strong, and vigorous right up until the time *they* decided it was time to die? In my opinion, the answer is totally, utterly, and absolutely *yes*!

Will you need to make changes to your diet and lifestyle if you want to live longer, happier, and healthier? Yes, of course you will. What are those choices worth to you? Will you have to totally sacrifice fast food, processed food, meat, dairy, wheat products, and alcohol that you currently consume on a daily basis? You can eat a healthier diet and consume some of those things occasionally as a treat. But if you want to live a happier, healthier life with lots of desire, energy, and vitality, your diet and lifestyle may need to change significantly. Do you need to make such radical changes? Only if you want to be around to see your children grow up, get married, and have your grandchildren. Only if you want to retire and still have enough glorious energy to go dancing, kayaking, skiing, hiking, and biking. Only if you want to take long, loving walks on the beach with your significant other, watch the sunset, and keep up with your grandchildren.

Not possible, you say? I say it's not only possible, but I'm living proof that you can do it. Thousands of other people are also proof it can be done, and you can do it too. I'm the evidence you can see, feel, and hear. You can change your life by changing how you look at things, starting with the food choices you make because that's where life begins.

It begins with what I call POP—the power of plants. This includes the vegetables in the produce section of your grocery store, at the local farmers' market down the street, at your local food cooperatives, or—if you have the land and the inclination—in your own garden. And now there are hydroponics and raised-bed gardens you can utilize right in your own backyard that are really easy to care for if you don't have the land or ground space for a sizeable vegetable garden. The volume of produce you can generate for a family of four from just one of these hydroponic or raised-bed planters makes the investment pay for itself in just a few short months.

Do you want to live vibrantly, take control of your life and the choices you make, and flourish? Or do you want to follow someone else's design plan for how you'll live and then wither away sooner than necessary? If you're making regular trips to the doctor for this or that ailment, this or that disease, only to have the doctor give you one prescription after another with serious side effects that can snowball into other malfunctions in your body, you're living someone else's design plan. This path can be slow, painful, and endless. I've seen it happen with family members and friends. I've also seen what other people like me have done to reclaim their health from near-death, stage-four, terminal cancers and other life-threatening diseases such as diabetes, heart disease, osteoporosis, and others. We've been resurrected! Yes, we've been resurrected from those near-death experiences to live and tell our stories. Can you do it? Absolutely, positively, the answer is *yes*.

We've been programmed to think that our ancestry or family history determines that we will succumb to certain diseases. Science has told us so, right? *Wrong!* Notice I use the word "programmed", because I believe that what we think gives birth to what happens to us in health as well as in life. If we believe the programming of our health is something we have no control over, then it is more likely that we will succumb to whatever disease or condition is part of our family history. This health impairment, this abnormal functioning of our body, becomes an expected part of our aging, so we look for it, even plan for it. You can avoid old family programming by changing what you eat, how you eat it, the kind of lifestyle you live, and your belief system.

You don't need to have a prizefighter's body with hard muscle mass and work out at the gym several hours a day, seven days a week, to be healthy and live a long time. However, you do need to move your body in gentle, loving ways every day. If you want an ocean of health, this book will show you how to get started.

So I ask you again, do you want to live, or do you want to die? If you answered, "Yes, I *want to live*," then let's get going. We have a lot to talk about. If not, you can start planning for the alternative.

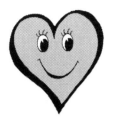

CHAPTER 2

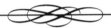

The Telling Mammogram and Diagnosis of Breast Cancer

IN ORDER TO MOVE FORWARD with my breast cancer recovery story, I want to take you through many of the details and processes that were precursors to my ultimate decision in choosing alternatives. These experiences affected me deeply—emotionally, physically, mentally, and spiritually.

My mother died from lung cancer when I was in my twenties. Seeing how traditional medical treatments affected her had a serious impact on my decision to use alternatives. I did not want to treat my cancer with conventional medicine. This story is also about how all these decisions can affect you, your family, and your friends. This level of detail will help you understand why I chose to use alternatives, how I believe I gave myself cancer, and why I can take it away. This important information may affect how you manage your own health care in the event of a diagnosis of any kind.

Life as Usual

I was having all my checkups, eating what I thought was a healthy diet; getting some exercise, having a cocktail now and then, and basically enjoying my life, my work, my family, and my friends. Then November 2004 rolled around, and it was time for my annual mammogram. Well, it wasn't so regular, because I was called back for a retake on December 23, just before Christmas.

The mammogram showed an abnormality, an unusual mass, in the left breast. It was not the first time this happened, and I was assured it was probably nothing, most likely just a benign cyst. However, the mass was in exactly the same location as the retake from the mammogram I had in May 2003, eighteen months earlier, which had revealed nothing unusual. They did a compression (ouch!) on the suspect area and decided *it* was nothing to be concerned about. Fast-forward to December 2004, and the *it* wasn't *nothing* this time; it was something that needed additional attention.

I actually looked at the mammograms (I had to see it for myself), comparing the last one taken in May 2003 and the one in December 2004. To my untrained eye, there was nothing I could see that showed any kind of mass, but I was advised to consult with my doctor about setting up an appointment with a surgeon for a biopsy. I wondered if there was actually anything there later. Many times when you see an X-ray of a broken bone, you clearly see the break or fracture. When someone has a tumor somewhere in the body, you can usually see it on the film. Even to the untrained eye, something should be visible, don't you think? Sometimes I wish I'd gotten a second opinion on the mammogram readings to better determine the small distinctions from one mammogram to the next. It just didn't feel right, not being able to see something on those films— trained eye or not. I suggest you do get a second opinion from a different hospital or health-care center if and when you ever have a questionable diagnosis.

So I went home that day feeling bewildered and called my gynecologist to see who he could recommend. I also called my general practitioner, who is an endocrinologist, to get a recommendation from him. After a round of telephone tag with each doctor, I came away with a name: Dr. Barbara. I proceeded to dial her number and made an appointment for a consultation in January 2005.

The days between December 23 and January 11 went by so slowly, snail like. It didn't matter that Christmas and New Years were in between with the regularly scheduled plethora of holiday festivities. I had a lot going on, so I was very busy but, as you might expect, deeply and emotionally distracted by the "what if" scenario.

When my mother died at fifty seven from lung cancer she was just seven years older than I was at the time of my diagnosis. She had the recommended standard treatment of chemotherapy and radiation. She also endured the expected side effects of vomiting and hair loss and was so weakened by all the treatments that she became bed ridden. My mother was a hairdresser, and it was just awful for her to lose her hair. Both my father and mother, when younger, were blessed with thick full heads of dark beautiful hair, now gray, and it was very emotional for me to see her lose hers.

I remember being told by my sister Joyce, who was there when my mother died, that my father said, "I wouldn't wish this on a dog." I had to give my dad a lot of credit, though. He and my sister Patti, and to a lesser extent my sister Joyce and I, took care of my mother on weekends at home, where she chose to die. She didn't want to be confined to a nursing home or hospital. I so bless my father for this now. It was hard on him and on all of us.

And here I was just seven years younger than my mother, at fifty years of age, hearing that I may have breast cancer. Needless to say, I was devastated and didn't quite know what to think, do, or expect.

Surgical Appointment

My appointment with Dr. Barbara was scheduled for January 11, 2005, at 1:30 p.m. Bill came with me, and I was not really concerned. I was healthy, so I was sure this cyst in my breast was going to be just that, a cyst and not a malignant tumor. We waited for what seemed like forever, and when we were finally escorted into the patient exam room, we waited some more. When the doctor finally came in, she explained all the details of the surgery and what it would involve and accomplish. How long the surgery would take, the anesthesia to be used, the lumps or indentations that would be left on my breast were just some of the infinite details she reviewed. The removal of tissue samples from the breast or any other part of the body apparently leaves an indentation in addition to a scar. This whole peculiar procedure was called a "biopsy with a needle localization." This "needle localization" didn't sound like it was going to feel good.

We left the doctor's office that day with an appointment for surgery first thing in the morning on January 25. I was given a host of information to review, along with pre-surgery instructions to follow and customary forms to fill out.

Day of Surgery—January 25

We showed up at the hospital at the required time and were escorted to the designated area for disrobing and redressing in those sterile hospital gowns that do so much to enhance your figure and cool you off. You know, they're short in length, just above the knee, and tie in the back but don't close completely. But this time I was instructed to put the gown on like a jacket, opening in the front. Obviously this was necessary because it was my boob that needed the surgery, not my butt!

In preparation for my surgery I was asked to remove all of my jewelry. Since I never wore much jewelry anyway, the only thing I had on was my wedding band and my engagement ring and a cross necklace. The additional thirty pounds I had put on in the last fifteen years almost caused my surgery to be rescheduled. I couldn't get my rings off! I spent a solid fifteen minutes running my ring finger and hand under cold water to reduce any swelling and soaped up my ring finger so the ring could more easily slide off. Finally, success. The thought of having to have my rings sawed off and having the surgery rescheduled for another day was not a pleasant one. The nurses had to make sure that anything that would restrict blood flow anywhere on my body was removed. The surgery would most likely cause my left arm, hand, fingers, and the area of the biopsy on my breast to swell.

Then I was moved via wheelchair back to the radiology department of the hospital for the needle localization. I was not to receive any anesthesia or numbing of my breast for this particular pre-operative procedure. I didn't like that idea but was assured it would just "pinch" a little. I would not experience any real discomfort or pain because there is so much fatty tissue in the breast. Apparently fatty tissue is not accompanied by nerve endings. *Ugh*! I was hoping they were certain about that because when I cut myself, it's painful, even for a minute or so. By the way, I'm fairly certain it must have been a male doctor who said sticking a needle deep into breast tissue was only going to pinch. Only a male could make such an assumption. Come here, Doc, let me put a needle in your breast and see how you like it!

I was situated in the same exam room where I had the last mammogram compression and was advised what to expect. When I saw the length of the stainless steel needle they were going to use to locate the suspected tumor area, I almost fell out of my chair. The nurse proceeded to place my breast in the crusher. You will know if you're a female and old enough to have had a mammogram what I'm describing here. This piece of radiology equipment squishes your soft breast tissue between two cold metal plates. Squishing is required. Making a pancake of your breast allows the radiation to reach deeper into the tissue and record what may be in there. In my case it was the suspect tumor.

The nurse told me I would have to wait a few seconds while she called another trained technician or doctor who would actually insert the needle. The purpose of this procedure is to provide the location of the tumor for the surgeon, just before the surgery. The technician looks at your X-ray while your breast is still in the crusher and then inserts the needle at the location of the tumor or cyst to be removed. This gives the surgeon a better idea from where to take the sample breast tissue. The tissue sample goes to the lab for examination and identification. This needle localization allows the surgeon to be more exacting in the tumor removal, lessens the duration of surgery, and shortens the time the patient must be under general anesthesia.

My breast was sufficiently squished, and the technician was summoned. It was a male doctor who didn't have much of a bedside manner, but then for the small part he played in my care that day, how much personality do you need to insert a long surgical stainless steel needle into a female breast? Curiously, why in hell wasn't the technician present at the very moment the breast was compressed, thereby eliminating the wait time necessary for him or her to be summoned? Doctors have more important things to do than wait for a breast to be crushed, so you are in a fairly high state of discomfort before she or he gets there to actually insert the needle.

The actual insertion of the needle into my breast took a couple of minutes at most, and much to my surprise I felt no discomfort or pain. I'm sure this procedure was painless because my breast was already numb from the crush and the time it took to summon the doctor who would insert the needle. The initial *pinch* that I was advised I would feel was indeed all that I felt. Once the needle penetrated the outer layers of skin, the doctor guided it into the suspect area without any pain via the technician's skilled hands. I guess there is something to be said for nerveless fatty tissue after all. The fear I was experiencing overcame any sense I had about such things anyway.

Once this procedure was over I was once again moved via wheelchair back up to the surgery waiting area, only this time, with an eight-inch needle sticking out of my breast. Now I was once again in the wait mode. After what seemed like an eternity the surgeon appeared with the anesthesiologist. Each one asked me at least three times my name, birth date, address, and if I knew why I was in the hospital. The surgeon then asked a few more times what breast she was going to biopsy. Then she marked the skin above the breast with a marker of some sort, and I was asked again if that was the breast that required the surgery. I guess the doctors and nurses do this in order to be certain they are doing the biopsy on the correct patient and the correct body part. I'm glad they do, yet I certainly would not have let the radiologist put an eight-inch needle into the wrong breast anyway!

After much anxiety and waiting, it was finally my turn. I remember being rolled out of the waiting area, saying good-bye to Bill, and rolling down the hallway into the operating room. The surgeon, anesthesiologist, and nurses were all with me. Once again I was asked who I was, why I was there, and which breast needed the surgery. The last thing I remember was the proverbial counting backward from ten. I never made it past five. I was *asleep.*

The anesthesia I was given was more than a local but less than a general, so when I woke up I felt as though I had just awakened from a good night's sleep. No hangover from the drugs, but having had nothing for breakfast in preparation for the surgery I was very hungry and wanted to leave. I was given a turkey sandwich and a can of ginger ale. I ate the sandwich and drank the ginger ale quickly, got up, got dressed, and left, but not before being given my instructions for postsurgical care. I was told to wear a sports bra for a few days and I could remove the bandages after twenty-four hours.

I felt fine; I really did. Bill dropped me off to pick up my car, which had some service work done on it that day. I drove home against doctor's orders and the recommended postsurgical procedures and care. Damn rebel!

We decided we weren't going to tell our sixteen-year-old son, Mike, about the surgery until we knew more about the outcome. An office visit was scheduled for one week after the surgery. We would discuss the results with him, if necessary, after the follow-up appointment. There was no point in upsetting him with a host of unknowns if we didn't need to. We were too upset and had no news to share at that point.

The days went by slowly, and I wondered what the biopsy would show. Why do patients have to wait so long for test results? This was not a simple, routine blood test to find out what my cholesterol level was. This could be cancer, and I wanted to know yesterday what the biopsy showed. There should have been some easy way to tell immediately what the scoop was. The emotional strain between surgery and getting any news at all is frightening, to say the least.

Follow-Up Appointment and Diagnosis—Breast Cancer

So here it was, seven days after the surgery, February 1, 2005. Our appointment was scheduled for 3:00 p.m. I was sitting at my home office desk around 2:00 p.m., waiting for Bill to come home so we could get to the doctor's office to learn the results. The phone rang, and it was my general practitioner, who is actually an endocrinologist I went to during my pregnancy with my son. I came down with gestational diabetes and carpel tunnel syndrome and was referred to him for care of the gestational diabetes piece.

Dr. Bob is a very nice, down-to-earth, personable guy who spoke most of the time in terms I could understand. He called to say he's sorry about the news. I asked, "What news?" And then he tried to do some fancy back tracking because he knew he let the cat out of the bag. There it was! I had breast cancer. Wow, what a way to find out, but is there ever a good way? And this is the reason patients should know immediately whether their biopsies or tumor removals are normal or not. Why the heck should all your doctors know it before you do? I guess they try to keep each other in the loop on patient care. It was *my* boob they took a sample of, why wasn't I in the *loop*? I told him we were on our way to see the surgeon for the lab report results at 3:00 p.m.

Was this God looking out for me, bracing me in advance for the news, or just a terrible twist of fate? Either way I was glad it happened because when the surgeon walked in and told us I just broke down and wept. Would it have been worse if I weren't forewarned? The surgeon told us that we should make an appointment with an oncologist to see what my options were. *Ugh!* What was next? There were so many unanswered questions, and this was just the beginning. The surgeon had a recommendation for two oncologists, even a favorite. I wrote down their names and numbers.

After dinner that night we told our son the news. He went into the living room to watch television, and I was surprised by his reaction, quite detached. He didn't have much, if anything, to say. I didn't know what he was thinking or feeling except over the next few days he was unusually kind. You know how teenagers can be. It seemed we didn't have any way of breaking through to what he might be thinking. Fear of losing a mother, was that it? What did he know of breast cancer and the ramifications at sixteen?

It wasn't until June 2012, when I was writing this book, that I decided to talk directly to him, now twenty-four, regarding his feelings about my diagnosis in January 2005. How incredibly insightful this conversation was more than seven years later.

Unclear Margins

The biopsy did indeed reveal a malignant tumor with cancer cells that had spread beyond the actual tumor to the far edges of the tissue samples. This confirmed that the cancer could have spread beyond the breast tissue and into the lymph system. This is known as unclear margins. Note that I said "tissue samples," as in the plural. They took two large samples of breast tissue from my left breast. After I reviewed the lab reports and saw how large the tissue samples actually were, I was stunned. I converted the centimeters to inches and drew two three dimensional rectangles on a piece of paper. Holy cow! How could they take what seemed like the entirety of my breast and still leave any left at all? I was a 34C in both breasts before the surgery and a 34B now in the left breast. By the way, the surgeon did a great job of going in to get the tissue samples. She went in just around the outer edge of the dark section of the breast known as the areola. There was literally no visible scar, just the dent she told me I would see, but even that was hardly visible. Thank you for that, Dr. Barbara.

Because the tissue samples indicated the cancer could have spread into my lymph system and beyond, my surgeon suggested an additional surgery called a *sentinel lymph-node biopsy* procedure. My surgeon also suggested surgically removing more breast tissue and some lymph nodes. Apparently this is helpful in diagnosing what stage breast cancer I had. It's also useful for determining how far the cancer had already spread from the tumor site into other parts of my body, particularly the lymph nodes around my breast and under my armpit.

This would help the doctors determine the course of treatment. Should radiation, chemotherapy and other drugs be administered? How much of each, how often, and for how long in an attempt to kill the cancer cells?

I left the surgeon's office after hearing the cancer diagnosis on February 1, 2005, with the sentinel-node surgery scheduled some time later that month. The surgeon who did the original biopsy and tumor removal would perform this surgery as well. In between the diagnostic office visit and the pre-surgical office visit for the sentinel node procedure I developed a long list of questions and questions-within-questions for Dr. Barbara to answer.

Oncology Visit

The surgeon suggested I make an appointment with an oncologist in order to discuss my treatment options. I did. I saw the surgeon's *favorite* in between the first and second scheduled surgery. What an eye opener that was.

Bill came with me to the hospital, where the oncologist had his office. The whole setup there looked very sterile and institutional. The sight of hospital worker's quickly moving all about with charts in their hands and gurneys carrying people with IV's of saline solution or blood in them just coming from or going to some test or surgery was highly sobering. We found our way to the oncologist's office, went in, checked in, and guess what? We waited. I was on time; where was he?

When it was finally our turn, we went into the examining room, and the doctor came in and introduced himself. Nice guy, personable—those were my first thoughts about this man. I was asked to take my shirt and bra off so he could examine me. He did. He performed the usual breast exam that a regular doctor would do as part of a routine annual physical. This time it wasn't routine. He was looking for lumps and bumps that would lead him to order more tests and X-rays, whatever he needed, so he could understand just what he was dealing with in my body. Bill later said it felt weird for him to be there as he watched another man, doctor or not, *feel me up*. Oh well, that's what it was like for him. For me it wasn't anything like that. Getting felt up usually has some sort of positive, sensual, heightened emotion attached to it. There was nothing sensual about this experience. It was downright intrusive—necessary, but intrusive. Once the doctor's hand had examined every inch of my body, he was finished, and I was allowed to get dressed. We then sat down, all three of us, and the oncologist said he noticed no obvious lumps or bumps during his examination of my body. That was good. We talked.

He began to explain all the different treatment options available to me and the scientifically-arrived-at success rates for using this radiation, that chemotherapy, this drug, and that procedure. Hmmm … here I was, about to become one of the statistics that could be referred to as a success or failure in the world of medicine. Wow, what an honor.

Radiation Therapy

According to medical wisdom at the time, if I chose to incorporate radiation therapy my cure rate would, of course, be higher than if I had none. My oncologist presented some percentages that I wrote down, all very confusing. I was playing the numbers game with my breasts and my body. The side effects of radiation therapy were redness and burning of the skin, killing cells that weren't cancerous around the target area, and possibly feeling tired.

Wait a minute. Isn't my heart in the center of my chest, in between both breasts? If the radiation was going to kill off cancer cells as well as cells in the surrounding area, what about my heart? What about the cells that make up my heart? Would they be hit with a dose of radiation, too? *You have to be kidding me*, I kept saying to myself.

Radiation that can kill cancer cells can also kill good cells, burn skin, and cause fatigue and listlessness. The best thing about radiation was that it was short term, a few weeks, maybe a couple of months. This would be administered four to five times a week. What a drag.

Tamoxifen

Tamoxifen was one of the chemotherapy drugs prescribed for stage one or two cancer patients at the time. The results from the second surgery would determine which cancer stage I was actually experiencing and the oncologist could then decide if tamoxfen was a drug to consider in my course of treatment.

The oncologist got very specific about the possible use of tamoxifen, a hormone therapy drug used to block the estrogen hormone. Excess estrogen has been shown to cause cancer, and it appeared my type of cancer was estrogen positive, which meant it would be receptive to tamoxifen. It could be taken orally in pill form for the recommended five years. Its side effects could be hot flashes; possible phlebitis, which is inflammation of the veins, usually in the lungs and legs; internal bleeding from the uterus; and uterine cancer.

I wasn't ready for instant menopause and hot flashes. If I did experience hot flashes, what prescription would he suggest to deal with them? Another drug!

I could experience phlebitis—swollen veins, usually in the lungs and legs. What about my lungs? I needed them to breathe. What about my legs? I needed them to walk, run, play, and dance. What were they going to do when my lungs got inflamed? Take them out, too? What about the other parts of my body? Weren't there veins in other parts of my body? How could this drug just affect the veins in my lungs and legs without having it affect the other veins in other parts of my body? What would happen if my brain got inflamed? What drug would you use for treatment of inflamed brain veins? What side effects would that drug cause?

Then there was the uterine bleeding and uterine cancer problem. Ok, so I take tamoxifen, and I start bleeding from the uterus. Is this a sign of uterine cancer? If not, what is used to treat a bleeding uterus when you aren't having your period? What do we do with the uterine cancer if I get that? Remove the tumors one by one until I have no uterus left? He said I may be required to have a total hysterectomy, another surgery to remove yet another body part. *You've got to be kidding me,* I said to myself again, again, and again.

Let me see. You take a breast cancer patient and give them a toxic drug to reduce the production of a hormone so cancer cells won't proliferate in the breast. In the process of trying to eliminate one disease, another is created in another part of the body, in this case my uterus. This drug ends up destroying a perfectly good healthy reproductive organ by trying to cure another part of the body.

I've got a perfectly good working uterus now. Why on earth would I compromise it by choosing this drug to treat my breast cancer? Then I would have to take yet another drug, hormone replacement therapy, for the rest of my life. The uterus does provide many hormonal benefits to women as they get older, even though they've passed child-bearing years and no longer have their period. I didn't like this motion picture at all.

Lupron

With this option I could take an injection every three months, and, like tamoxifen, it would turn off the estrogen production but could cause profound hot flashes and related symptoms.

Other Tests

My oncologist wanted to be sure I didn't have tumors growing in other parts of my body, so he ordered a round of more familiar tests to take before my next surgery. They were a bone scan, chest X-ray, MRI, and a cat scan. These seemed all fairly harmless, except the chest X-ray, with the additional dose of radiation. My breasts had already been exposed to three in the past couple of months. I wasn't a fan of this at all, but it seemed logical for a complete set of diagnostics to be done, so I went along with all of the additional tests.

Oncology Summary and Guinea Pig

Helloooooo ooouuuttt theeerrreee! Is anybody listening? Does any of this make any sense to you? What about any of this was good and in my best interest? All I could see was cut, burn, or poison in all of the recommended treatments.

I began to feel like a medical guinea pig, a hamster on his exercise wheel. I kept running and running and running and I wasn't getting anywhere, except tired and worn out. I couldn't get off, couldn't stop. There was nowhere to go. It seemed I could become medically dependent on the never-ending cycle of taking one drug after another to fix one thing that could cause multiple system failures in other areas of my body. It seemed they were recommending, under the guise of medical knowledge, the creation of one harmful condition after another and maybe never getting rid of the one that initiated all of this.

There were so many questions about *what if* scenarios that really none of them could be answered in advance of the second surgery. Once the data were in, my life and my future could be foretold by my team of medical experts. Sounds like a Superbowl event doesn't it—my team? Who will win, and who will lose? Everyone is working hard for me, right? My team, knowing the full extent of just how far the cancer had spread into my breasts, my lymph node system, and/or other parts of my body, would be able to then make more educated guesses as to my course of treatment.

Once the second surgery had been performed and the results were in, the oncologist would have the necessary information to suggest the appropriate treatment(s), how much, and how often.

Pathology Report

The pathology report revealed the tumor to be 1.2 centimeters, or equal to just under one-half inch in size. That would make me a stage one or two cancer patient. The tumor was definitely considered stage one. The second surgery I was scheduled to have would reveal if any further cancer cells in the lymph nodes were present. If no cancer cells were found, I was a stage-one cancer patient. If they found more cancer cells, then I would be classified a stage-two cancer patient.

Second Surgery, Pre-Surgery Office Visit

During a sentinel-node surgery a surgeon injects a dye into the diseased breast through the breast nipple. This dye is supposed to follow a path that somehow the cancer cells would have taken and will identify which lymph nodes and additional tissue samples to remove for biopsy.

I guess that made sense. Yet I wondered, if this procedure was so important, why didn't they do this sentinel-node procedure with the first surgery? I suspect that if the tissue samples had clean margins, meaning no cancer cells around the outer margins, the surgeon could feel safe in knowing they *got it all.* Keep in mind that I already had two large chunks of breast tissue removed. The largest tissue sample was 6 x 4 x 2.5 centimeters. The second tissue sample was 3 x 2 x 1.8 centimeters. For those of us still on the inches and feet scale, let me rephrase this. The first sample was approximately 2 ¼ x 1 ½ x 1 inches and the second tissue sample was approximately 1 ¼ x ¾ x ¾ inches. If you draw this out on a piece of paper, you'll see just how large these tissue samples were. Now I admit that I'm using a rectangle shaped box to draw these dimensions out on paper, and the lab technician in the pathology department was probably using the widest, longest, and deepest portions of the sample, but still. Oh my goodness! These samples were huge!

I may have been a busty 34C in both breasts before the first surgery, but after the tissue samples were removed from my left breast I can say with certainty my left boob is now a 34B. In addition to that, I can clearly see that my right breast hangs a little lower than the left breast. (I guess I now know how guys feel, but at least they don't wear a bra on their testicles, except if they play sports requiring cups.)

Much to my surprise this did not cause me any bra-buying problems. I decided not to wear one any longer anyway. I wore mostly underwire bras, which I've since learned cut off blood circulation and create drainage problems for your lymph system around your breast and armpit areas. This can generates a storehouse of trapped toxins that could become cancerous over time. No surprise here.

The answer my surgeon gave me to the most important question I had for her just blew me away. This was in preparation for the second surgery. Hear ye, hear ye, come all and hear ye! Please pay close attention to this scenario.

Try to imagine this. You have a big maple tree that generates sap for making maple syrup. You cut the tree down and then remove a large section from the trunk. So you're left with the trunk section rooted into the ground and the sectioned off piece with the limbs and leaves still on it, the middle section gone. Then you try to reconstruct the tree by putting the top cut portion of the tree back on top of the remaining stump still rooted to the ground. Do you think the sap is going to go up the tree the same way it would have if it weren't cut? I don't think so.

The conversation with my surgeon went something like this:

"Dr. Barbara, you've already removed two very large breast tissue samples from my breast, one sample containing the tumor. Hasn't the original path and pattern of the capillaries within the breast been redirected now because of this removal? The internal flow of the blood and lymph fluid is different now that some tissue is missing and internal scarring has taken place. How do you know the dye will flow to the lymph nodes that would have been affected, with the tissue that was there now missing? How can this procedure identify the exact location of the cancerous lymph nodes and other cancerous tissue within the breast now that the integrity of the breast tissue has been compromised?"

She looked at me with a straight face and said, "Well, Linda, that's a very good question."

I didn't get an answer that made any sense.

That was my first turning point away from conventional medical treatment. I felt if the surgeon performing my surgery couldn't answer what I thought was a simple question, and she thought it was a good question to ask, there was no way I was about to succumb to the knife a second time.

I'm sure many people just trust their doctor completely for solutions and answers, but I saw my mother go through that type of programming and wanted, so far, no part of it.

I went home from that appointment with a renewed sense of dedication and conviction to find another solution. None of these proposed *solutions* sounded safe, effective, long lasting, or pleasant to deal with. They also came with so many side effects and didn't seem to really deal with the cause of why I got cancer in the first place.

Research of alternative solutions brought me to information on the use of organic raw foods. The nutrient density of specifically green vegetables was very powerful in rebuilding your immune system. Eating a raw-food diet was beginning to look *great*! Sure sounded a lot less invasive, painless, and had plenty of wonderful side effects, none of which involved vomiting, burning my skin, more surgery, or additional body part removal. An incredibly healthy body, that's a side effect worth working towards.

Use of Thermography in Place of Mammograms

When it's time for your next regularly scheduled mammogram, you may want to consider replacing mammography with thermography. There has been some research to suggest that mammograms could possibly be an actual cause of breast cancer and spread it as well. Considering how uncomfortable a mammogram is anyway, if there is another option, then why on earth not use it?

If you ever choose to get a mammogram and are told you need a *retake*, I would ask for breast thermography instead. This procedure is totally noninvasive and painless. All you do is stand in front of a camera. There is no breast pain experienced by the squishing of the breast between two metal plates and the exposure to yet another dose of radiation. Thermography is a heat-sensitive test. When you have inflammation of any kind, anywhere in your body, the inflamed area is hotter than the rest. So, in the event of a cancerous tumor or other kinds of inflammation in your body, there's a good chance thermography will pick up the tumor faster than the X-ray and with no additional radiation exposure or side effects. Love it!

Doctor Calvin Ross is a certified X-ray technician who clearly has many concerns about the use of mammograms and details the reasons why at his website. Dr. Ross states that "Mammograms were introduced in 1965 and just four years later in 1969 the first report appeared stating X-ray radiation was causing breast cancer." Just four little years after the use of mammograms there was an indication that breast X-rays (radiation) were causing cancer. Then why hasn't the use of this technology been stopped? Was it the medical equipment manufacturer's investment in the technology, equipment, and training that pre-empted the decision to thwart any legitimate concerns this report may have presented? (drrossdc.com. 2013)

If I sound harsh and bitter from this experience, I was. I now had breast cancer. Where did I go from there?

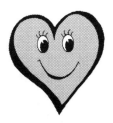

CHAPTER 3

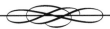

Decision Time

I LEFT THE DOCTOR'S OFFICE THAT day with a renewed sense of independence; there had to be another way. No longer did I think traditional options were my only choices, yet I still wasn't sure which direction to take. I still wasn't absolutely convinced, so the next phase of my journey involved more research.

Research, Research, Research

There is so much information out there on the Internet and in print for researching everything, and breast cancer was no exception.

I read dozens of books on the effects of drugs, chemotherapy, and radiation—both the good and bad. I then tried to understand the double-blind studies that purportedly confirmed beyond a reasonable doubt that these drugs and methods were safe, in spite of the deadly-sounding side effects.

I found the courage to research everything about my particular type of breast cancer. I asked for all of the test result reports from every doctor, surgeon, radiologist, or technician who was involved in my care. I began to research all the medical terms included on the reports so I could better understand just what they were actually saying, and if I didn't know the layman's translation after looking up all those words in dictionaries, I asked.

Don't be shy. It's your body they're going to cut, burn, or poison, and you have every right to know just what every single word means in these reports and how those words will affect the doctors' decisions on the care they recommend to you. Then it will be your decision how to allow them to care for you. Ask for copies of all your mammograms, ultra sounds, chest X-rays, body scans, bone scans, and the initial diagnostic-biopsy report. Put these things together and try to tell your own story of what's going on in your body. Pay particular attention to how you're feeling as you read all these things and the effect this information has on your *gut reaction*.

My *favorite* new website became breastcancer.org. I learned a ton about my diagnosis on that site and am so grateful for all the information it provided. The website had pictures of *infiltrating-ductal carcinoma*, my official diagnosis on the pathology report. It was wonderful to literally see, through pictures, what was actually going on inside my breast and how this cancer could spread. (BREASTCANCER.ORG "IDC – Invasive Ductal Carcinoma" 2013) The information presented on that site was also written in very clear, understandable language. Thank you to those behind the scenes at breastcancer.org. (BREASTCANCER.ORG 2013)

Both of my nieces worked in the medical field. One is a physical therapist and the other had a nursing degree and was working in the radiology department of a local hospital. The radiologist described at length how radiation could benefit me. The newer technology was better at targeting a specific cancer area. I was glad to hear that, as I was concerned the radiation was going to kill good cells around or in my heart along with the cancer cells. This information made me more comfortable in accepting the side effects of burned, reddened skin, as well as the swelling, and the killing of good cells would be minimized. Is killing good cells along with the bad really a good thing in any treatment scenario? I think not. That didn't feel good, and it didn't feel right.

My other niece was well-versed in the technology also, and between the two of them I was feeling less concerned about the radiation part of the treatment, if that turned out to be my intended direction. Still, I was not convinced.

My research also included reading articles on ways to overcome cancer and other diseases with diet, vitamin and mineral supplements, and detoxification. We absorb many toxins from the processed food we eat, municipal water supplies, the air we breathe, and common household and beauty products. Many of us aren't even aware these toxins exist and have no idea what effect they can have on us. Our body doesn't recognize what to do with these toxins because they aren't part of the body's biochemical makeup, so instead of being processed out through normal channels like the blood, liver, bowel, and urine, they get stuck. Another form of toxicity comes from the amalgam fillings in our dental work. Amalgam fillings generally contain heavy metals like mercury, silver, and gold and were never meant to become part of our body, anywhere.

I became captivated by all the information I was seeing and reading on the body's ability to heal itself through simple yet effective ways. I was beginning to become intrigued by the power of plants. Raw food, fresh fruit and vegetable juices, green smoothies, moderate exercise, and vitamin and mineral supplements cleanse the body from the inside out and rebuild the immune system.

I thought, *I have to eat anyway, so why not eat the food that's going to make me well?*

The best thing about these alternatives was that they came without harmful and deadly side effects. Not one of them indicated I would get a secondary disease, illness, or symptom if I took them. Only good and wonderful things would happen. My body would become whole and healthy again. And the parts that were not diseased but not operating at peak efficiency, well, those would become healthier, too. The alternative ways of healing became much more interesting as my research continued. Health is everything, and if you truly are what you eat and the diet and lifestyle I had before cancer caused me to become sick, then my diet needed changing.

Dr. Lorraine Day

I watched a number of videos and television infomercials, and a few in particular began to stand out and make a great deal of sense. My research focused for quite a while on Dr. Lorraine Day's website. Dr. Day is an internationally acclaimed orthopedic trauma surgeon and best-selling author. She was on the faculty of the University of California, San Francisco, School of Medicine as associate professor and vice chair of the Department of Orthopedics for fifteen years. She was also chief of orthopedic surgery at San Francisco General Hospital and is recognized worldwide as an AIDS expert. She was diagnosed with late-stage breast cancer twenty years ago and is still working full-time and taking part in all the activities she enjoyed in her twenties. She looks absolutely gorgeous at seventy-five. See her pictures on her website, along with a wonderful, vast multitude of healing information. (Day 2013)

I eagerly studied her personal breast-cancer recovery story during which she used alternatives almost exclusively. Her protruding tumor extended several inches from between her breasts in the middle of her chest. She decided to have some of it surgically removed to make it easier for her to get around but refused all other types of traditional treatment. You can read about her recovery and what it took and see for yourself how as a medical doctor and surgeon she refused standard medical treatments recommended by her oncology colleagues.

Dr. Day's videos started to make a really big impact on me, and her website was so incredibly comprehensive it could be a one-stop-shopping location for alternative health information. I certainly don't recommend this, however, because everyone has different needs. You should really do your own research to see what rings true for you but it's definitely a stop on the dial. She refused chemotherapy and radiation even though she is a surgeon. Watching how she shared her in-depth experiences with breast cancer and her subsequent recovery made incredible sense to me. At one point she said she didn't get cancer from radiation, chemotherapy, or other drugs, so how could using those tools be successful in eliminating the cancer? Well, that made perfect sense to me. What *was* the real cause?

A Cancer Battle Plan

My sister, Patti, reminded me of a book called *A Cancer Battle Plan* written by Anne E. Frahm with David J. Frahm, which was about Anne's alternative recovery from breast cancer in 1990. After an initial misdiagnosis, Anne was diagnosed with stage-four breast cancer. After a year of conventional cancer treatments, including chemotherapy, radiation, bone-marrow transplants, and blood transfusions, she was sent home to die and given five to eight weeks to live. She and her husband Dave refused to give up, prayed for an answer, and then received a book from a friend about the link between nutrition and cancer. They sought out a good nutritionist; Anne rebuilt her immune system and lived several more years before she died in 1998. But she didn't die from cancer. She died from iron toxicity that shut down her liver, resulting from the many blood transfusions she was given during the bone-marrow transplants. When she died, the doctors didn't exactly know what she died from until they did an autopsy. It was another senseless death caused by the use of modern medical so-called treatments. She died from an iron-poisoned liver caused by the blood transfusions and not the cancer. So, in effect, she died from the treatment! (Frahm and Frahm 1992)

Natural Cures "They" Don't Want You To Know About by Kevin Trudeau

Then there was Kevin Trudeau. I watched as he was interviewed on an early-morning television show talking about his book, *Natural Cures "They" Don't Want You To Know About*. As a consumer advocate, Trudeau exposed many government offices, pharmaceutical companies, and food manufacturing companies for their greed and corruption in their desire to produce and manufacture *food* that was making us sick. This information paralleled other information I'd read on the Internet that was basically saying the same thing. Cures for cancer were already out there, but people were being silenced and paid to keep quiet about them. Is this a free country? Is this the United States of America, the land of the free and the brave? Why on earth was the cure for a disease like cancer being swept under the carpet or being held in a closet behind locked doors? I began to feel like I stepped into a suspense and drama film based on conspiracy and deception. Could any of this be true? Not in my country. I was in for a huge awakening. (Trudeau 2004)

I was aware of the controversy surrounding Kevin Trudeau. The next day I went to the bookstore and bought his book. I was devastated, alarmed, and dismayed at the information I read. Trudeau talked about processed and dead food, as well as the perils of MSG, aspartame, high-fructose corn syrup, hydrogenated vegetable oils, sugar, natural and artificial flavors, and spices. Artificial flavors and spices are just a myriad of chemical compounds bound together to form a food additive that's highly addictive, makes food taste great, and is completely devoid of any nutrition. My spice cupboard was filled with artificial sweeteners I thought were a great substitute for calorie-rich sugar. Little did I know the chemical makeup of this sweetener or the long-term effects it could have on my body. I have more to say on this subject later.

The information in Trudeau's book sounded a lot like other information I read from other sources, with little or no controversy about the authors. I was treading lightly, but I couldn't help feeling there was a lot of truth in his words. The many books I later read from reliable sources confirmed everything—*everything*—I read in Trudeau's book.

He painted a dismal picture of our government, the health-care system, farming, and food processing in America. He had nothing good to say about anything he shared. My eyes and my mind were beginning to open, and I didn't like what was I was seeing or feeling. Believe it or not, I was actually beginning to understand how diet and lifestyle can cause a variety of illnesses and diseases, not just cancer. There was so much information out there confirming this that it had to be true. There was also a lot of information on how to get rid of cancer and diseases of all kinds with food, vitamin supplements, detoxification, and meditation.

I was way off track from what I thought was a healthy diet and lifestyle. Just repeating what I learned growing up 'didn't make it right or healthy. It just made it what I learned growing up. An open mind could possibly improve your life. A closed mind could cause you to shrivel up and die, emotionally, physically, mentally, and spiritually.

I was often awake in the middle of the night with my mind reeling from trying to process too much data, and my red, bloodshot eyes wouldn't shut long enough to go to sleep, so, late night and early-morning television got what little energy I had left. I felt numb most days after all the processing. The sleepless nights were beginning to wear on me, but I kept up the pace. I felt there was something larger than life to be discovered and it was going to affect me in profound ways.

Naturopathic Doctor, Friend, and Fellow Curler

It happened because I was in the right place at the right time. I had been curling for a few years and met some wonderful people. Yes, the sport called curling is now an official winter Olympic sport, a sport that's played on a bowling alley-like sheet of ice using forty-two pound, polished-granite stones. A broom is used to sweep in front of the stone as it moves down the ice toward the other end. I curled and loved it!

I learned that one of my fellow curlers was just finishing up her program of study to become a naturopathic doctor. A naturopathic doctor and a medical doctor train the same way, up to a point. They both go through an intense study of human anatomy, but when it comes time to learn how to treat disease and illness, there is a parting of the ways. Medical doctors go on to train in how to use surgery and drugs to treat the symptoms of disease and illness, with varying degrees of toxic side effects. Naturopathic doctors seek to understand the underlying causes of disease, thereby suggesting changes in diet, lifestyle, and detoxification that will contribute to a lifetime of wellness.

Most often alternative options or treatments are noninvasive and have no unpleasant side effects. There is no cutting, burning, or poisoning in this practice. Alternative options like vitamin and mineral supplements, herbs, mild exercise, meditation, yoga, and detoxification are good for the whole body, strengthening and rebuilding the immune system so the disease goes away. The whole body gets well, not just the diseased area.

When I discussed my diagnosis with my naturopathic curler friend I couldn't believe what she was telling me. She confirmed all the information I had been collecting from various sources about the body's innate ability to heal itself. We just need to give it the tools it needs—raw fruits and vegetables with live enzymes, moderate exercise, and good sleep—and steer clear of chemicals of all kinds at all costs. She gave me a detailed sketch of how our cells get sick, explaining free radicals and what they do in our body to create sick cells that could grow out of control and become cancerous tumors. She also believed there were many natural cures for cancer that had been covered up in order to keep the medical, drug, and health-care industries alive. After all, without sick people there wouldn't be the need for so many doctors, pharmaceutical companies' toxic drugs, or health-care facilities and workers.

Cassette Tape (Remember Those?)

Another friend of mine who was also interested in health care traveled a lot. He let me borrow a cassette tape recording of a doctor in California who was coaching a female patient to avoid breast-cancer surgery. She followed this doctor's advice, opted not to have the surgery, rebuilt her immune system, and recovered from the cancer. She was grateful for the coaching. Again, this doctor talked about the same things already discussed above.

There was a pattern developing. A vivid picture was beginning to take shape, and it didn't involve the *traditional* medical community.

Decision Time

The amount of information I was attempting to absorb from conventional and alternative treatment options caused me to feel stifled and overwhelmed. Trying to understand and digest all of it times felt insurmountable, like undertaking a climb of Mt. Everest without any training. At this point I still hadn't decided which path of treatment I wanted to use—alternative therapies or traditional medical treatments. I spent many sleepless nights praying to God for help in making the decision that would restore my health, no matter which one it was.

Then it happened. One night, after I had concentrated on, contemplated, and condensed about as much information as I could take, it happened. I lay in bed wide awake, eyes looking straight up to the heavens, again mulling over the chemotherapy option and remembering the side effects my mother went through.

I asked and begged God, "Please give me some kind of sign to know which direction I should take."

Ask and you shall receive. My God and my angels were with me. There it was! The answer came to me just as clearly as I know my own name. The light bulb went on! My inner vision painted this vivid picture of a big yellow smiley face, only it wasn't smiling. That big, welcoming yellow circle we're all familiar with that usually wears a wide, friendly smile had a big old frown on it. That was it! I was convinced this symbol was the answer to my prayerful pleading. The frowning smiley came to me as I considered chemotherapy. This was the symbol I asked for.

God said, "No, don't go there!"

With that I decided to embark upon a plan my doctors could not and would not condone. I chose to use alternatives.

Canceling Surgery and Notifying My Oncologist

After I decided to use alternatives, I needed to do a few things. First, I needed to cancel the sentinel-node biopsy procedure as it was just around the corner. When I called to cancel the surgery I initially spoke to the nurse, who asked if I was sure I wanted to cancel and tried to convince me to keep my appointment. I said thanks, but I had made my decision, and I could sense a wall of fear well up in the nurse on my behalf.

I then called the oncologist's office. Of course, I didn't get a chance to speak directly with the doctor right away, so I left a message through his nurse or receptionist telling him also of my plans.

That same afternoon I got two calls, one right after the other. The first one was from my surgeon, urging me again to follow through with the surgery as she reminded me of the consequences of my actions. While she was not happy about my decision, there was nothing she could say or do to convince me to move forward with that sentinel-node procedure: die injected into my breast through my nipple and sent on a journey to find cancerous lymph nodes. No way, Jose! Raw food sounded a whole lot less invasive, not to mention healthier.

The second call was from my actual oncologist, not a nurse or secretary. He was also very concerned. When I explained to him all I had learned about the impact of a raw-food diet, rebuilding my immune system and changing my lifestyle, the only thing he could respond with was, "Well, this is all I know," and we ended our phone conversation. I actually felt a little sad for him because he really did sound sincere. He left me with the impression that maybe he knew the treatments he trained for and was offering weren't working for his patients.

Think about the amount of time, money, education, and training needed to become a doctor. Then add a specialty like oncology on top of that, and what you have is one heck of a bright woman or man with a lot of technical and medical information stored in their memory banks. To think of the skill and ability needed to practice medicine simply boggles my mind.

I'm sure the oncologist's ego took a big hit, too. Imagine, someone like me, a woman untrained in the wonders of cancer treatment in the United States of America, making a decision to go against conventional medicine, wisdom, and training.

Suck it up doc. I respect what you do, but this is my body and I will decide what to put in it or on it, who touches it, and how I will manage my disease called breast cancer. There I was, thinking for myself. I was off the beaten path, outside the box, pushing the edge of the envelope and making decisions about the direction of my own health care that made sense to me. Imagine that!

I thought if Dr. Lorraine Day and Anne Frahm could recover from their late-stage breast cancers, I could certainly do it at stage one or two. What did they have that I didn't have? Nothing! We're all valuable people, no matter what our backgrounds, and part of making any decision like this is recognizing your own value. I was beginning to see mine.

Summary

Think about this for a minute and see if it doesn't make sense to you. If you cut yourself with a knife while chopping up some tomatoes—what happens? You go *Ouch* and see the physical cut; it most likely starts to bleed a bit, and you run for a bandage. These are symptoms of the cut. What next? Well, the first thing you do is stop cutting yourself. Sounds silly, but it's true. You don't continue to cut the cut in order to heal from it.

If you eat a plethora of processed foods, salty and fatty snacks, and a gallon of ice cream every single night after dinner, chances are you're going to be very sick—if not now, later. What are the symptoms of obesity? There are many, not the least of which is being overweight, maybe diabetic, discomfort, sleeplessness, and lethargy. You don't look very good and probably have a hard time enjoying making love with your partner, if you have one. What do you do to lose weight? What do you do to regain your health? You stop eating all those processed foods, salty and fatty snacks, and a gallon of ice cream every night after dinner and begin an exercise routine, among other things.

You don't continue to use the object that cut you or made you obese to begin with in order to heal your cut or to lose weight.

If you eat junk and other foods that are lifeless and you are diagnosed with cancer, diabetes, heart disease, or something else, then what do you think you should do? Stop eating those lifeless foods and replace them with foods that are vibrantly filled with the nutrition your body is starved for and craving. The net result is the cut heals. You lose weight. You get healthy and cure your disease.

If I didn't get cancer by using chemotherapy, radiation, or surgery, what makes me think I can get rid of it by using these same treatments? The body knows what it needs. Listen to it. Listen to it very carefully and seek out some alternative-care providers who can help you understand your own body's language.

CHAPTER 4

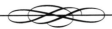

HealthQuarters Ministries

Finding the Right Place

After researching a number of different alternative health support facilities, both locally in and around the Northeast and all across the United States, I decided to go to a place in Colorado Springs called HealthQuarters Ministries. (HealthQuarters Ministries 2013)

HealthQuarters was started by Anne and David Frahm after Anne's recovery from her near death experience with stage-four breast cancer. David Frahm went back to school and became a naturopathic doctor, a master herbalist, and a certified nutritionist. HealthQuarters Ministries continues now under Dr. Frahm's guidance.

Trying to find the right place to get some alternative care was not really that difficult, partly because there just weren't that many choices, and the basis of recovery was always the same—raw food and raw juices, immune system strengthening, detoxification, supplementation, and spirituality. One facility was in Massachusetts, one in New York City, a couple in Florida, some in California, and some even in other parts of the world.

I made notes on each one and then called to interview them over the phone, as much as humanly possible under the circumstances. The length of stay and the type of programs offered at these facilities all varied. The costs varied widely, too, from a few thousand to tens of thousands or more, plus traveling expenses. Something about HealthQuarters in Colorado Springs stood out among the crowd. So HealthQuarters it was.

Once I got there I understood why. It was the people and the place. This facility was an attractive and comfortable old-style motor inn. There were small cabins that Dr. Dave and his team had turned into lovely guest suites, each with its own character and décor, making the lodge, as they called it, more like a fine bed and breakfast. The lodge was located at the base of the Garden of the Gods, and there was a certain spiritual energy I felt about the whole area of Colorado Springs. The staff was well informed, kind, compassionate and supportive. I was supposed to be there.

My sister Patti came with me to offer support, even though she was well. Who but a sister would offer to come with me and go through this experience when I was the one who was sick? We shared a lovely two-bedroom suite with just one bathroom. This made it difficult when it came time for our twice-a-day water and coffee enemas, but the lodge provided a schedule, we worked it out and had fun anyway. Yes, we had fun. There was no television or radio in the room, just peace and quiet. The whole experience was just wonderful.

The Physical Program and Related Education

The damage done to the immune system and other systems from improper and excessive bad fats, regular table salt, white sugar, tobacco, alcohol, and prescription drugs, along with too much cooked food, is a recipe for disaster. But enzyme-rich, fresh-made fruit and vegetable juices help heal every cell in the body of the damage done by consuming a diet of revolting excesses.

The program was all about getting my immune system back into shape in order to regain my health. The plan involved doing a fast for eight days, but not the kind you may think. This program was called a juice fast, and we drank only liquids during the first five days. Over the last two days we were slowly introduced to solid food again in the form of soups and salads.

We consumed freshly made juices and a host of vitamin, mineral, and herbal supplements. While these supplements were optional, they were also highly recommended. I took a colon cleanser and did a parasite cleanse. I took a powdered drink mix to help detoxify my liver. We gave ourselves coffee and water enemas and a liver/gallbladder flush.

I drank half of my body weight in ounces of fresh, pure water each day to continually flush my system of toxic wastes that were being released from the cells in my body. When cells start to regenerate with the good stuff, the bad stuff has to go somewhere. It gets dumped into the lymph and blood system, so continually drinking plenty of fresh, pure water is important. We did some rebounding and gentle walking to keep our systems flowing. A couple of ladies trained in foot and body massage gave us those luxurious treatments, as well. These were some of the amazing things we did and learned about. I needed to rebuild my seriously malfunctioning immune system, and it needed all the help I could give it.

Educational classes offered during the day presented detailed information on the effects of clean water, clean air, organic food, and the detox surprises we may experience while there. Moderate exercise is also a part of the program. I learned about a three-foot-wide mini trampoline called a rebounder that you can slowly and gently jump up and down on to help your lymph system drain from toxic build up. Without movement, toxins get stuck, backed up, and then can become a target area for disease. That's one of the reasons why exercise of any kind is so important. I took many leisurely walks in the Garden of the Gods, as I enjoyed the surrounding beauty and contemplated my return to health.

That phrase "no pain, no gain" is a lot of crap! You don't have to pump iron and exercise until you experience pain or feel like vomiting in order to stay healthy, unless you want to get sick. Pain equals stress, and stress is just not good for the body under any circumstances, whether physical, emotional, spiritual, or otherwise; unless, of course, you need to run like hell for your life. Under those circumstances a certain amount of stress is good. It's called the "fight or flight syndrome."

I was amazed at what I learned about diet, toxicity, exercise, stress, and how and why the body revolts when it doesn't get what it needs. HealthQuarters presented this information in an incredibly articulate, concise, and comprehensive way. I was a sponge, and I couldn't soak up enough of this information. I was devastated to think I was fifty years old and hearing most of this information for the first time in my life. It was filling a void I didn't know existed. The education and the detoxification, well, they were the parts that would hook me for life.

The loving, peaceful, and nurturing environment of HealthQuarters Ministries provided just the right atmosphere I needed to get away from all the stress that led up to this trip. The people were warm and sympathetic and knew each and every one of us could overcome our disease with the right tools, the right attitude, and a desire to live. I'd never known or experienced such a complete feeling of love and support at any time in my life, especially from complete strangers. When it came time to go home, I cried. I didn't want to leave this encouraging and nurturing place or the people who had been caring for us during the previous eight days. The education they gave us, the feeling and emotional connection they shared, and the care and concern they demonstrated were just wonderful. I didn't want it to end.

The Political Education

That peace and calm I felt wasn't going to last long, though. I didn't know that once again I was going to be overwhelmed with more information. This time, though, I was going to get mad, really mad—madder than I remember being in a long time. I knew I wasn't supposed to get the hair up on the back of my neck, but I did. I was about to learn things that made me feel I had been living under a rock for the last fifty years.

We received intense health and wellness education about things in our environment that could contribute to cancer. Some are polluted air and water, the containers in which food is packaged, and the conditions under which some animal farming is done. I was overwhelmed. Again, my eyes and ears were opening for the first time, and I didn't like what I was seeing or hearing. I learned that our government, the pharmaceutical industry, and our health-care system guard information that can make us well, all in the name of corporate greed and profits. I became angry when I heard this, and, more importantly, it's happening right under our noses and most of us don't even know, or care about it.

I can actually reverse cancer on my own. Do you understand the power of that statement? I can actually reverse cancer on my own. *My body is that perfect and powerful*, and so is yours. There are government leaders and corporations that want nothing to do with us getting well by using food and vitamin supplements. They have products, pills, and potions to sell us, as they reap huge billion dollar profits. This is garbage, and it's a part of what our health-care system is comprised of right now.

Every single person who said *yes* to alternatives and said *no* to traditional medicine knows this. We are thousands strong, and we are making a difference!

Summary

I came to understand that disease is caused by a severely weakened immune system. Consuming poor quality or dead food, breathing in poor quality air, drinking poor quality water, and choosing a really bad lifestyle can do incredible harm to our bodies. Conversely, consuming high quality, organic, live foods; breathing fresh, clean air; drinking pure water; and making better choices about our work, our family, and our health will contribute to a vital, enduring, healthy body, mind, and spirit.

To continue the program at home I was instructed to do a monthly seven-day fast, like the one outlined above, for up to a year. My diet became organic vegetarian, although carnivores who just can't give up animal protein could add organic chicken, turkey, or wild salmon periodically. I discovered I felt better when I didn't consume animal protein, so my diet consisted of 80 percent raw fruits and vegetables and 20 percent cooked foods. Freshly made organic juices, made by using a juice extractor of some kind, are huge when trying to overcome an illness. I continued to drink at least five glasses of various kinds of freshly made vegetable juices every day. I ate lots and lots of green vegetables and some fresh fruit.

It felt great knowing I was in charge of my body regaining its health. I was in a grateful state of appreciation to think I didn't have to go through the traditional medical treatments that would cause me to lose my hair, vomit, and be tired all the time, not to mention burning my skin with radiation and undergoing more surgery. I was not only excited, I was in ecstasy! I felt like this was the only answer and I was going to give it all I had, and I did.

I couldn't believe the positive side effects of this program. Seeing these side effects made a definite believer out of me. When I saw the physical evidence in the form of impacted fecal matter, candida yeast build up, and cholesterol deposits that showed themselves from the enemas and liver/gall bladder flushes just during the eight-day stay at HealthQuarters, I was absolutely convinced we do give ourselves cancer.

I Gave Myself Cancer, and I Can Take It Away!

The healing had begun. Each one of us is responsible for our own health; we're in charge, completely and totally in control of our health and to what extent we want to thrive, not just survive.

Thank You God, Thank You God, and Thank You God for steering me in the direction that was best suited for me.

Please go to the HealthQuarters website and watch three short YouTube videos from Dr. Dave Frahm and his beautiful late wife, Anne, in which they share their passion about health, Anne's diagnosis, and her program of recovery from breast cancer.

CHAPTER 5

What Is Disease and What Causes It?

THE FIRST THING ABOUT GETTING well was coming to a realization of what I was doing that wasn't working. Breast cancer—just what was I doing that I didn't understand about my diet and lifestyle that caused breast cancer? I was doing a lot wrong. In this chapter I will share what I learned from a variety of sources about what can cause cancer and other diseases. In the next chapter we'll talk about what I corrected and how I reformed my lifestyle to become cancer free and whole again.

While I mention many toxic chemicals and other contaminants that can paralyze and sabotage our bodies, I'm only going to review some of them here—those, I believe, that had a real impact on why I got cancer and how eliminating them stimulated my return to wellness.

What Is Disease?

Disease is an abnormal condition, a health impairment that contributes to improper functioning of the body. A disease can lead to serious illness or even death. If you are diagnosed with any disease chances are it is the result of a malfunctioning or failed immune system.

I've heard that broad definition repeatedly since attending HealthQuarters, and it makes a great deal of sense. Disease is not normal.

Cancer is not normal. Health is normal, and if your immune system is in tip-top shape, there is no reason you would ever develop any disease, cancer, or other illness.

So what is an immune system? By definition the word "immune" means exempt, resistant, and unaffected. The immune system, then, is the body's protective mechanism for preventing disease and illness. If it's strong, then you will not get sick.

Traditional medical treatments only *mask* the symptoms of disease, while alternative solutions get down to the source of the problem so you can eliminate the root cause, thereby creating ultimate healing and infinite wellness.

That's what we want to do, right? Treat the source of the problem and eliminate it. We don't want to put a sheet over the symptoms and say, "There, symptoms gone; problem solved," do we? We want to get to the bottom of the cause so we can eliminate the disease for good. That is the main difference between traditional and alternative medicine. This made incredible sense to me after all I'd been reading. But still, what caused *me* to get breast cancer? It's the immune system that isn't functioning properly, or none of us would ever get sick. Your immune system gets sick; therefore, you get sick.

Disease is not a by-product of old age, either, unless you abuse your body, your diet, and your lifestyle your whole life. The medical profession just loves to say this ailment or that ailment is the result of growing old or from a genetically passed down predisposition to disease. Well, yes, that may be true, if the diet and lifestyle you've chosen or been handed through generations creates toxic buildup in both your mind and body. Your body and mind will get sick, but they don't have to; there is a better way!

My Copper Toxicity Regarding Old Age

I saw a nutritionist while I was going through the detox phase of my wellness plan, and I used her guidance and services as a marker for how I was progressing. After we talked for a bit she noticed a brown spot on the right side of my face about the size of a nickel. She asked if I had that on previous visits. I said yes and that I didn't know where it came from. It wasn't causing me any pain or discomfort, and it wasn't a vanity issue for me, so I just ignored it.

Jokingly I asked her, "What's the cause of this brown spot, old age?"

"No," she said, "it could be an excess of copper in your system showing itself as those brown spots on your face."

Really? I was quite surprised to hear this. The spot on my face was the symptom; copper excess could be the cause.

She had some personal experience with copper poisoning when she was younger, and her medical doctors at the time had no idea what was causing her to be so lethargic, languid, and listless all the time. So she embarked on a quest of her own to find out what was happening to her. Sure enough, once she found someone who could test her for it, she had five times the amount of copper in her body than the average. Once she went through a copper detox plan she regained her strength, and her symptoms vanished. She used a diet plan than involved foods that had no, or very low, copper content.

She suggested I have a tissue analysis to measure my copper levels. For a tissue analysis a lock of hair is sent to a lab and broken down to determine what minerals are in the hair. Hair is considered a tissue and can be a dumping ground for excesses the body is trying to eliminate, not just copper. Sure enough, my tissue analysis showed I had about twice the normal range of copper in my body. Even though I didn't have the same symptoms as this nutritionist, I sure had the brown spot, smaller ones, too, in different places on my body.

We went through a whole list of foods and beverages I was consuming that could have contributed to this spot, and we found several. Even as a raw foodie, I was eating foods I didn't know were high in copper content. Dried fruits and nuts in particular are high in copper. It didn't matter that I was consuming predominantly all organic fruits and vegetables; the copper is a natural part of the fruit or nut. I proceeded to eliminate those dried fruits and nuts and other things she suggested, and true to form, the spot started to melt away. My nutritionist suggested I read *Why Am I Always*

So Tired? by Ann Louise Gittleman, Ph.D. with Melisssa Diane Smith. The entire book is dedicated to copper excess and what to do about it. (Gittleman and Smith 1999)

Many traditional medical doctors call these brown spots "aging spots," and everyone gets them as they get older. I believe that everyone gets them because many people consume a lot of coffee and tea, and those liquids are naturally high in copper, too. I certainly drank my share. My nutritionist also mentioned that prescription drugs contain many heavy metals, and copper is one of them. Since more than fifty percent of adults aged fifty-seven to eighty-five rely on five or more prescription drugs each day, is it any wonder age spots are showing up on their skin? Is it any surprise that people get *age spots* as they age?

I found it amazing to see ads on TV for products that are meant to fade *unsightly* brown age spots. I later learned these products contain a bleach-like ingredient, which gives them the ability to fade the brown spots. So is that a cure or a cover up?

Old age? I don't think so anymore. Our country needs many more naturopathic doctors, nutritionists, and others like them to reach the underlying cause of disease and not just cover up the symptoms.

I was absorbing all this information like a sponge. The more you know, the more you want to know.

Cause of Breast Cancer

From experience, the naturopathic doctors at HealthQuarters shared what they believed to be a repeated pattern of nutritional deficiencies that lead to breast cancer. The same six areas came up every time, and I was no exception. I had a weak thyroid, liver, and colon; unbalanced estrogen; and a shortage of zinc and essential fatty acids.

How do they know this? Many naturopathic doctors and other holistic health-care practitioners use a system called muscle response testing, or MRT, which is also commonly known as biofeedback or kinesiology. Every organ and tissue in the body produces and emits an energy pattern, and there are certain points, like acupuncture points, on the body where these organs can be tested. The doctor or practitioner assesses the body's need for various nutrients like vitamins, minerals, amino acids, and essential fatty acids using MRT.

Then the practitioner reaches into his or her toolbox of supplements and muscle tests that supplement with the client. This helps identify which nutrient would be best for correcting this imbalance and how much of the nutrient would be required to bring the body back into balance again.

Because of our varied diets and lifestyle stressors, the nutrients in the body may be used up when tested today, but when tested again next week can be sufficient. For example, if you have an MRT test today, and your body indicates a shortage of vitamin B12, the practitioner will put some vitamin B12 into your hand, adding as many tablets or capsules as necessary until your body tests strong for vitamin B12. You then take the recommended dosage for the recommended amount of time. When you go back to get retested in a few weeks or months, your body may test normal or strong. Your practitioner may suggest either reducing or eliminating the supplement for a while until the next test.

Once you're on a healthier diet and you get most of the nutrients you need from your diet of raw organic fruits and vegetables, your need for supplements may lessen or could be eliminated altogether.

What These Systems Do

I'm sure everyone remembers that childhood song about bones: the toe bone's connected to the foot bone, the foot bone's connected to the ankle bone, the ankle bone's connected to the leg bone, etc., right? Well we might as well rephrase it to go something like this. The thyroid is connected to the liver, and the liver is connected to the colon, and the colon is connected to estrogen, and estrogen is connected to zinc and essential fatty acids.

These systems are all interdependent and muscle response testing, repeatedly, showed them to be malfunctioning or inoperative in breast-cancer patients. When one system is out of balance it can have a snowball effect on the rest of the organs and systems in the body. This pattern may play a big role in whether or not you fall prey to breast cancer. Dr. Dave

Frahm from HealthQuarters and author of *The Breast Cancer Pattern, It Starts With Your Starving Thyroid* describes the process. Here, in my words, are just a few of his findings. (Frahm 2009)

Low Thyroid Function

The thyroid produces hormones that run the energy production in every cell of the body. The thyroid runs on iodine, and our Standard American Diet provides basically no iodine. Don't be fooled into thinking you're getting iodine in regular table salt; you're not. Unless you're taking an iodine supplement of some sort or eating a seaweed-rich diet, you're probably not getting enough iodine to keep your thyroid running smoothly.

Congested Liver Function

Our liver gets its energy for detoxing the body from the thyroid, and the liver is responsible for breaking down excess estrogen and removing it from the body. What happens when anything gets congested or plugged up? It stops working.

Did you ever have to change the filter on your heating or air-conditioning systems? Those 12 x 16 x 1 inch filters that get so clogged up your HVAC system can't breathe? Well, your liver is no different. Many of your organs are meant to process or purify some system in your body, and when your organs are abused by bad food and beverage choices, they just give up. They just don't work as efficiently, if at all, any more.

Sluggish Colon

The colon also gets its energy from the thyroid and is responsible for flushing out of the body what the liver removes from the blood. When both the liver and the colon are plugged up, congested, or sluggish, toxic wastes, including excess estrogen, are stored in the fat cells of the body. Most fat cells are generally found in the breast tissue of most females.

Unbalanced Estrogen

The female body must always have progesterone in balance with estrogen at a rate of ten times more progesterone than estrogen. When your thyroid isn't operating at peak efficiency, it can lead to the buildup of estrogen in the breast tissue. Because of the highly refined, carbohydrate-filled Standard American Diet, the female body is inclined to menstruate without ovulating. When ovulation does not occur, progesterone is not produced, which can stimulate the growth of breast, uterine, and ovarian cancers.

Zinc and Essential Fatty Acids Depletion

When estrogen dominates, zinc supplies are exhausted. Zinc is important for the proper functioning of the immune system along with a host of other functions.

When zinc stores are diminished, essential fatty acids are not absorbed well, and they are vital to the healing of injured cells and the production of healthy new cells.

Okay, but I still wondered what causes these nutritional deficiencies to occur and why I was also deficient in these areas. Seems my diet was beginning to become a major-league player in why I got breast cancer.

What Are Disease Contributors?

There are hundreds, if not thousands, of different toxic-disease contributors. First and foremost is our food supply, as it has become purposely contaminated and injected with fillers and addictive additives like MSG, aspartame, and many more. Other disease contributors include household cleaning products; laundry detergents; fabric softeners; chemically-based fertilizers, pesticides, herbicides, and fungicides; chemical food additives; personal-care products like makeup, perfumes, and colognes; food preservatives; toxic air and water; environmental stress; physical, mental, and emotional stress; cookware coated with plastic; plastic wraps used to store food; electromagnetic energy fields; microwaves; exhaust fumes from automobiles; and the beat goes on.

Unless you're working in a factory-like setting and getting exposed to a barrage of chemicals every day, in my opinion our food supply probably has the largest toxic load of disease contributors, and our conventional and processed food supply is practically void of any nutrients. Oh, there are plenty of ingredients, but where's the nutrition? And if there are any listed on the labels of packaged and processed products, there's a good chance the package indicates that some of these vitamins have been added back in. Where did they go that they need to be added back in? During the processing all the vitamins and minerals were cooked out, squeezed out, or washed out. That's processed food. Let's take a look at some toxic disease contributors.

Toxic Food

The Standard American Diet—animal protein, hydrogenated and saturated fats, sugar, salt, caffeine, refined processed food, dairy products, cooked foods, soda, diet soda, and junk food— are just some of the foods we consume that are creating diseases in our bodies.

All of these standard food items in our fridge, pantry, and freezer are acid-causing foods. Our blood needs to be 7.365 pH, or slightly more alkaline than acid. When we consume more acid-causing foods than alkaline foods, our enzyme stores become depleted, and we need enzymes to live. There is a complete chapter later in this book on enzymes, what they do, where we get them, and what life would be like without them. It's enough to say right now that we can literally not breathe or live without enzymes. (Ph In Balance 2010)

Soda

Phosphoric acid may interfere with the body's ability to use calcium, which can lead to osteoporosis or softening of the teeth and bones. Phosphoric acid also neutralizes the hydrochloric acid in the stomach, which can interfere with digestion, which makes it difficult to utilize nutrients.

Soft drink manufacturers are one of the largest users of refined sugar in the United States. It's a proven fact that sugar increases insulin levels, which can lead to high blood pressure, high cholesterol, heart disease, diabetes, weight gain, premature aging, and many more negative side effects. Most sodas include over 100 percent of the Recommended Daily Allowance

(RDA) of sugar. An average ten teaspoons of sugar are contained in each can of regular soda.

Diet Soda

Aspartame is a chemical used as a sugar substitute in diet soda. There are over ninety-two different health side effects associated with aspartame consumption, including brain tumors, birth defects, diabetes, emotional disorders, epilepsy, and seizures. Further, when aspartame is stored for long periods of time or kept in warm areas, it changes to methanol, an alcohol that converts to formaldehyde and formic acid, which are known carcinogens. (SweetPoison.com 2010)

Doritos, Oreos, and MSG

When I was growing up, all through elementary, middle, and high school, my favorite after-school snacks were always Doritos or Oreos, sometimes both. It wasn't just a few tortilla chips, loaded with salt, fat, and artificial cheese and chemical additives, but half or sometimes the whole bag. We're not talking small individual size bags here. We're talking the *big* ones. The Oreos were not just an afternoon snack with a couple of cookies and a small glass of milk before dinner, but a whole sleeve of them down one side of the bag.

How much fat and sugar, more *dead food,* can any one person consume before it takes its toll? I also wasn't a particularly active kid. Yes, I rode my bike, played roly-poly, weeded the garden, and swam occasionally, but I preferred TV to any of those more active kid things. Saturday morning cartoons were the best. Well, the body can in fact take a lot, because I was relatively healthy, or thought I was, until my breast cancer diagnosis on February 1, 2005.

Your body doesn't just one day wake and say, "I'm going to give myself cancer today," and, presto, you're sick! It's a long process that's the accumulation and culmination of everything you eat and drink, feel, say and think. Our bodies, over a lifetime, become the presentation of whom we chose to become. Then one day your body gives a wake-up call and starts screaming, *"I can't take it anymore!"* and you've just been diagnosed with some brand-name disease. Pick one: arteriosclerosis, different cancer types, diabetes, arthritis, osteoporosis, and lupus are just a few. It's the result, for many of us, of a lifetime of harmful eating and drinking. Let's add to that the consumption of a plethora of over- the-counter drugs, pharmaceutical drugs, and body products loaded with toxic chemicals. Let's also add to that formula having a pessimistic attitude toward life and harboring negative emotions and destructive feelings. No wonder you're sick with some kind of disease. Now you have another label, a disease you can talk about.

Sugar and fat consumption in this country is staggering. Go into any grocery store, local pharmacy, package store, or gas station and you'll find nothing but junk food at the check-out and for much of the space in every direction, all screaming *Buy me! Buy me!* The sugar, fat, chemical additives, and especially my favorite called *natural flavorings or natural spices* are shouting at you, loudly! And these unhealthy snacks are cheap. I'll bet you can't eat just one. I couldn't. I had to have two, three, or more servings, and really, what is a serving anyway, just a few chips or a couple of cookies? Who has the willpower to *eat just one*? Especially now that the candy-bar and individual-serving package sizes are so much smaller than when I grew up. It takes more to make you feel like you've had any at all. It really drives me crazy to see the words *all natural* on many products. What a short sell. I could stir up a batch of mud, add some fat and sugar to make it real tasty, shape it into cookies, add some *natural flavoring*, and call them *all natural*. I'll bet someone would buy them, and like them.

Sugar and fat-laden processed-food products are even more addictive now that *natural spices and natural flavorings* are routinely added. What are these, you ask? They are just a different form of MSG and serve to enhance the flavor and addict you to many canned and processed food products by excessively stimulating your taste buds.

I suggest you purchase the book or watch the YouTube segment by the same title "Excitotoxins: The Taste That Kills" so you can read or hear Dr. Russell Blaylock share his depth of knowledge about excitotoxins. Please, understand the impact this information could have on your health and that of your babies, children, and the rest of your family and friends. (Blaylock 1997) or (Blaylock 2011)

MSG is an amino acid, which is a by-product of a protein that was thought to be safe because it came from nature. Food manufacturers aren't required to list MSG on a food ingredient label unless it's 99 percent pure or more. Many people think it's the sodium in the MSG that's the problem, but it's not; it's actually the glutamate.

Dr. Blaylock is a respected, nationally recognized, board-certified neurosurgeon, health practitioner, author, and lecturer. He has more than twenty-five years of medical experience and is not afraid to dispute organizational thinking. He doesn't parrot claims by the *New England Journal of Medicine,* which receives heavy subsidies in advertisements.

Natural flavorings and spices, along with all the other additives listed below, according to Blaylock are versions of MSG. These flavorings are highly addictive, and because they're added to just about everything in our processed food supply, they are difficult to completely eliminate unless you're consuming a 100 percent organic, unprocessed-food diet.

During World War II Japanese soldiers were captured by American forces, along with Japanese rations. It was discovered that the Japanese rations tasted much better than those of our American soldiers. Why? The American Quartermaster Corps learned that MSG is a derivative of a natural ocean-grown seaweed called *kombu,* and the Japanese used this to enhance the flavor of food for over 1,000 years, most recently in processed canned rations.

Glutamate is the natural flavor enhancer. These flavor enhancers like *natural flavors* or *natural spices* can kill off thousands of brain cells, perhaps damaging the brain, and are highly addictive. Because these additives are addictive, people eat more and more of the processed food that contains them. Highly processed foods that contain many different MSG ingredient forms can be high in fat and salt, and virtually void of any nutritional content. Because these products are void of any nutrients, the body is never satisfied. You end up eating yourself to death by starving your body along the way.

If you haven't noticed, I have some hard core resistance about MSG and all its subtitled names disguised to seem harmless.

Food manufacturers in the United States were having problems keeping processed food tasting good, so they listened closely when the American Quartermaster Corps discovered the flavor enhancing properties of MSG and called a meeting to discuss it. Blaylock also said that "MSG allowed the processed food to taste better and last longer, so you can imagine the dollar signs these companies were visualizing at the time." (YouTube "Excitotoxins: The Taste That Kills" 2013)

This is the part that really gets me going. Baby food manufacturers began adding MSG to all levels of baby food, including infant formula. When they were made aware of the damaging effects of MSG, they voluntarily took it out of level-one baby food products; however, they kept it in all other levels. MSG is now a billion dollar business, and is it any wonder it's in everything processed?

What this means is that our children—no, our babies—are being given this addictive, brain-cell-killing substance before they even have a chance to learn for themselves the negative life-threatening effects of this natural substance. Not everything that comes from nature is good for us. It saddens me to see the recent trend to sell more packaged and processed food by labeling products with words like *natural* or *nature made*, implying that because it came from Mother Earth it's safe to consume.

MSG and many of its other named forms is also prevalent in all kinds of canned, bottled, and frozen foods. No wonder they appear to taste so good.

You simply need to be more discerning and pay attention to the ingredient list on the box, can, or other container. If you buy milk, you want the ingredient list to be one: milk. You don't want the ingredients to be milk, milk solids, carageenan, fructose, etc. Hopefully you're buying raw organic foods of every kind including dairy products. Try to buy fresh organic fruits and vegetables, no labeling required there. You know what you're buying and eating. If you buy bananas, you know the only ingredient is banana. If you buy a fresh, raw, organic tomato, you know the only ingredient is a tomato. Packaged goods that say they're natural are not necessarily good or healthy for you. Now that you know about MSG, you can do a much better job at filling your grocery cart.

As Dr. Blaylock points out, humans are five to twenty times more sensitive to MSG than any other life form. Carageenan, another name for MSG, is highly inflammatory and is used as a homogenizing agent, generally in liquid beverages but also in other processed foods that require thickening. Some foods say they are MSG free, but may contain three, four, or more of any of the ingredients listed below.

In the community where I once lived I started a raw food club called Eating in the Raw. I showed the DVD equivalent of the YouTube video called "Excitotoxins: The Taste That Kills," which, of course, featured Dr. Blaylock speaking about excitotoxins. (YouTube "Excitotoxins: The Taste That Kills" 2013)

After watching the DVD several times before the actual meeting date, I went to the grocery store and purchased a variety of infant formula and baby food up through the junior age, along with a variety of familiar name brand soups—cream of mushroom, cream of celery, cream of chicken. I compared the ingredients with the lineup listed below and was truly discouraged and appalled to find so many from each column in just one jar, bottle, or can. These are addictive, cheap fillers and do nothing to feed your starving cells and organs, not to mention the need to nourish your babies' and toddlers' developing bodies.

This is primarily why I eat a raw organic fruit and vegetable diet. I know what I'm eating. No food processing or artificial addictive additives in these food items. When my stomach tells me I'm full, I know I'm full of real food nutrition, fiber, vitamins, and minerals that my body can recognize and assimilate to enhance my immune system and keep me well. I don't eat out much because there just aren't many raw food vegan or vegetarian restaurants around that can tempt my taste buds like I can with my own food preparation. I can add as much garlic, onion, and raw vegetables to a dish as I can muster up. I also make a lot of raw green smoothies and raw soups. No one wants to be around me for very long after one of those meals, with all the garlic, but, hey, I'll be around a lot longer than they will. I just *know* it!

I once went to a holistic fair, and a multilevel marketer was selling a *natural* vitamin that tasted like strawberries. Sure enough there was a *natural flavor* additive listed on the label. I asked the representative what this natural flavor was and he responded, its strawberry. I said I didn't think so or the label would have just said *strawberries* as the ingredient. And I'm very sorry to say this company is not alone. There are many multilevel marketing companies selling so-called healthy supplements where excitotoxins are listed ingredients. A multilevel marketing company is a business model in which independent distributors are compensated not only for their sales of a product or service to customers but also for sales made by other distributors they have brought into the company. (eHow "What Is Multi Level Marketing?" 2013)

Some multilevel marketing companies sell a jelly-like chewable they promote as a whole food supplement. This product is targeted toward children and these chewables are supposed to take the place of several servings of fruits and vegetables each day. Remember Juicy Fruit jellied candies? Well this product is like that, and it contains *natural flavors*. When these manufacturing companies get young folks hooked and addicted at a young age, you get them for life, right? I was literally shocked when I saw this, but I was assured this company was not going to do anything to compromise the health of younger children. Well, the company is a very large one, and I would rather put my faith and trust in the study and research of Dr. Russell Blaylock, a neurosurgeon, than a large company looking to obtain its market share.

Information provided by the Truth in Labeling Campaign provides evidence of just how many different names there are for diluted versions of MSG. Some individual food ingredients, when combined, can actually create MSG. Oh my!

Some people get reactions after eating the food ingredient monosodium glutamate, reactions that include migraine headaches, upset stomach, fuzzy thinking, diarrhea, heart irregularities, asthma, and mood swings. What many don't know is that more than forty different ingredients contain the chemical in monosodium glutamate (processed free glutamic acid) that cause these reactions.

The following list of ingredients that contain processed free glutamic acid has been compiled over the last twenty years from consumers' reports of adverse reactions and information provided by manufacturers and food technologists.

Names of Common Ingredients that Contain Processed Free Glutamic Acid (MSG)[1]
or
Create MSG During Processing

Names of ingredients that **always** contain processed free glutamic acid:	Names of ingredients that **often** contain or produce processed free glutamic acid during processing:	The following are ingredients suspected of containing or creating sufficient processed free glutamic acid to serve as MSG-reaction triggers in **HIGHLY SENSITIVE people:**
Glutamic acid (E 620)[2]		
Glutamate (E 620)		
Monosodium glutamate (E 621)	Carrageenan (E 407)	
Monopotassium glutamate (E 622)	Bouillon and broth	Corn starch
Calcium glutamate (E 623)	Stock	Corn syrup
Monoammonium glutamate (E 624)	Any "flavors" or "flavoring"	Modified food starch
Magnesium glutamate (E 625)	Maltodextrin	Lipolyzed butter fat
Natrium glutamate	Citric acid, Citrate (E 330)	Dextrose
Anything "hydrolyzed"	Anything "ultra-pasteurized"	Rice syrup
Any "hydrolyzed protein"	Barley malt	Brown rice syrup
Calcium caseinate, Sodium caseinate	Pectin (E 440)	Milk powder
Yeast extract	Malt extract	Reduced fat milk (skim; 1%; 2%)
Yeast food, Yeast nutrient	Seasonings	most things low fat or no fat
Autolyzed yeast		anything Enriched
Gelatin		anything Vitamin enriched
Textured protein		anything Pasteurized
Whey protein		Annatto
Whey protein concentrate		Vinegar
Whey protein isolate		Balsamic vinegar
Soy protein		
Soy protein concentrate		
Soy protein isolate		Amino acid chelate
Anything "protein"		
Anything "protein fortified"		
Soy sauce		Citrate, aspartate, and
Soy sauce extract		glutamate used as chelating
Protease		agents with mineral
Anything "enzyme modified"		supplements.
Anything containing "enzymes"		
Anything "fermented"		
Vetsin		
Ajinomoto		
Umami		
(1) Glutamic acid found in **unadulterated protein** does not cause adverse reactions. To cause adverse reactions, the glutamic acid must have been processed/manufactured or come from protein that has been fermented.		
(2) E numbers are use in Europe in place of food additive names.		

Reminders

Low-fat and no-fat milk products often include milk solids that contain MSG, and many dairy products contain carrageenan, guar gum, and/or locust-bean gum. Low fat and no fat versions of ice cream and cheese may not be as obvious as yogurt, milk, cream, cream cheese, cottage cheese, etc., but they are not exceptions.

Protein powders contain glutamic acid, which, invariably, will be processed free-glutamic acid (MSG). Individual amino acids are not always listed on labels of protein powders.

At present there is an FDA requirement to include the protein source when listing hydrolyzed-protein products on labels of processed foods. Examples are hydrolyzed-soy protein, hydrolyzed-wheat protein, hydrolyzed pea protein, hydrolyzed whey protein, hydrolyzed, corn protein. If a tomato, for example, were whole, it would be identified as a tomato. Calling an ingredient tomato protein indicates that the tomato has been hydrolyzed, at least in part, and that processed free-glutamic acid (MSG) is present.

Disodium guanylate and disodium inosinate are relatively expensive food additives that work synergistically with inexpensive MSG. Their use suggests that the product has MSG in it. They would probably not be used as food additives if there were no MSG present.

MSG reactions have been reported from soaps, shampoos, hair conditioners, and cosmetics where MSG is hidden in ingredients with names that include the words "hydrolyzed," "amino acids," and/or "protein." Most sun block creams and insect repellents also contain MSG.

Drinks, candy, and chewing gum are potential sources of hidden MSG and/or aspartame, neotame, and AminoSweet (the new name for aspartame). Aspartic acid, found in neotame, aspartame (NutraSweet), and AminoSweet, ordinarily causes MSG type reactions in MSG sensitive people. (It would appear that calling aspartame "AminoSweet" is the industry's method of choice for hiding aspartame.) We have not seen neotame used widely in the United States.

Aspartame will be found in some medications, including children's medications. For questions about the ingredients in pharmaceuticals, check with your pharmacist and/or read the product inserts for the names of "other" or "inert" ingredients.

Binders and fillers for medications, nutrients, and supplements, both prescription and non-prescription, enteral feeding materials, and some fluids administered intravenously in hospitals, may contain MSG.

According to the manufacturer, Varivax–Merck chicken pox vaccine (Varicella Virus Live), contains L-monosodium glutamate and hydrolyzed gelatin, both of which contain processed free-glutamic acid (MSG) which causes brain lesions in young laboratory animals, and causes endocrine disturbances like *obesity* and *reproductive* disorders later in life. It would appear that most, if not all, live virus vaccines contain some ingredients that contains MSG.

Reactions to MSG are dose related, that is, some people react to even very small amounts. MSG-induced reactions may occur immediately after ingestion or after as much as forty-eight hours. The time lapse between ingestion and reaction is typically the same each time for a particular individual who ingests an amount of MSG that exceeds his or her individual tolerance level.

Remember: by food industry definition, all MSG is "naturally occurring." "Natural" doesn't mean safe. "Natural" only means that the ingredient started out in nature, like arsenic and hydrochloric acid.

Information provided by the Truth in Labeling Campaign
Web: www.truthinlabeling.org
Phone: 858-481-9333. e-mail: adandjack@aol.com

Look at all these additives that go into processed foods. Pretty amazing, isn't it? And when you think of all the processed foods available for quick sale and a quick meal, whether you're eating fast, microwavable, oven-ready, canned, or bottled processed foods, you start to recognize the overall glutamate consumption in any given day. You can easily see why you can become addicted to processed foods. And if that isn't enough, check out your waistline and your general state of health and see what's happening there. (truthinlabeling.org "Names of ingredients that contain processed free glutamic acid (MSG)" 2013)

I recently went to two rather large family gatherings. I sat there and looked around at between thirty and forty people at each party, and I couldn't believe what I was seeing: severe obesity. The fire alarm went off. It was a reminder and wake-up call to finish this book as quickly as possible because these folks were young parents, and aunts, uncles, and grandparents of small children. Afraid to be in the sun, they all huddled around shade trees, not interacting with these beautiful youngsters.

What are their diets, lifestyles, and lives about to allow their bodies to get this out of shape so early in their lives, at such a young age? What will their children's health be like as they grow older? I can tell you for certain, they will be addicted to a junk food diet. Junk, diet, and processed foods are taking a toll, a huge toll. These foods are so easy aren't they? What's the long term cost of *easy*?

Animal Protein and Digesting It

Whether you believe in eating animal protein or not for humane and/or environmental reasons is unimportant and irrelevant for this example. We're just going to focus on the consumption of animal protein and what it does to your body.

Dr. T. Colin Campbell, Ph.D. authored a book with Thomas M. Campbell II called *The China Study*. Their book was the culmination of a twenty-year partnership of Cornell University, Oxford University, and the Chinese Academy of Preventive Medicine. (Campbell and Campbell 2005)

The research indicated that two groups of rats were fed a highly toxic cancer-causing substance called aflatoxin. One group was fed a diet of 20 percent protein, while the other was fed a diet of 5 percent protein. Every single animal that was fed the 20 percent protein had evidence of liver cancer. Every single animal that was fed the 5 percent protein avoided cancer. Nutrition overcame the carcinogen in a low-protein diet. It was found also that the protein casein, which makes up 87 percent of cow's milk, contributed to all stages of cancer development.

The study noted: "In fact, dietary protein proved to be so powerful in its effect that we could turn on and turn off cancer growth simply by changing the level consumed." The safer proteins were from plants. A big *wow*, please! (Campbell and Campbell 2005, 6)

This twenty-year-plus scientific research study is evidence that animal protein in the presence of powerful carcinogens can possibly influence the growth of cancer and other diseases. And by contrast, a 95 percent plant-based diet can prevent the occurrence of cancer, and further, can reverse cancer. I'm evidence of that, as are so many other alternative cancer survivors.

See the chapter on testimonials from several people who have used alternatives to cure themselves of cancer and other diseases. Most no longer eat meat at all, but if they do, it is in that 5 percent range that Dr. Campbell discussed. The meat is organically grown without bovine-growth hormones, grass-fed to slaughter, and no chemicals are used in the processing.

Toxic Water

In chapter 22 on Air and Water Purification Strategies, Dr. Frahm states "Drinking from the tap is like shooting your self in the proverbial foot." says Dr. Dave Frahm in his book *A Cancer Battle Plan Sourcebook*. (Frahm 2000, 164)

Regular tap water in America is filled with toxic chemicals, chlorine, and hundreds of trace pharmaceutical drugs. The chemical fertilizers, pesticides, and fungicides used in conventional farming, on golf courses, and on our lawns aren't all absorbed by the plants. The runoff seeps into the ground and eventually becomes part of our water supply. If you're not taking pharmaceutical drugs for any specific condition and drinking regular tap water, you are consuming pharmaceutical drugs anyway. Yes, in reduced dosages, but they are still finding their way into your body through a contaminated water supply. How does this happen? When those people who take these drugs use the bathroom for urinating or bowel movements, the excess is deposited into the water supply by way of sewage treatment plants, etc. Even though the water is chemically treated with chlorine to kill the bacteria and filtered, it's still not pure water.

If you live in a municipality that's required to give an annual drinking water quality report to all the residents, what do you do with it when you get it? When I get mine, I look at it and see pages of chemicals and toxins in *trace* quantities that some government agency somewhere has determined are safe for human consumption. Really?

Toxic Air

You all know the difference between air that smells sweet and clean and air that doesn't. Have you ever been to or lived in a very large metropolitan city and then taken a vacation to the mountains or to the beach just to feel the impact of the air quality when you got there? Even growing up in a small town—Bennington, Vermont—I noticed an air quality difference when I went further into the mountains. Why is this? The trees and all vegetation breathe in carbon dioxide and exhale oxygen, while humans breathe in oxygen and exhale carbon dioxide. What a beautiful life-sustaining system Mother Nature gave us. But when the system gets off balance, the home, the city, the state, and the country gets sick. The air gets so thickly polluted with toxic chemicals that we can't breathe. You've all seen news clips of big cities during the day. Los Angeles comes to mind, and I'm not picking on LA here. The smog is so thick sometimes you can't see very far.

The problem is that there is a shortage of trees and plants now, and the air cleanup process they perform quite naturally cannot be done effectively any longer. There just aren't enough green plants or trees to restore the natural balance.

When our bodies take in excessive amounts of toxic air, what do they do with all those toxins? Where do they go in our bodies when they can't be filtered out? Our lungs and liver are already plugged up from other things, primarily the dead food we consume, so they can't help either.

Check out the US Air Quality Map for your state among others. Seems we have a really big job to do at cleaning up air quality all over the United States. (Creative Methods 2013)

Self-Induced Toxic Lifestyle – All Stressors to the Body

Microwaves actually change the molecular structure of the food warmed or cooked in them. Don't use them as they alter the food quality and can cause cancer. (Natural News.com "Why and how microwave cooking causes cancer" 2013) Smoking, alcohol consumption, drugs and medications, breast implants, unnecessary plastic surgery, mammography, poor sleep habits, lack of exercise, artificial hormone replacement therapy, and emotional stress are some other self-induced toxic lifestyle stressors.

I suggest these items listed above are self-induced because we absolutely positively without a doubt have control over them. It's no surprise to any of us any longer how all of these body stressors just pile up. What does our body do with them when we have only so much filtering capacity? Disease is the net result.

Other Toxic Products

Fluoride toothpaste, laundry detergents, fabric softeners, cleaning chemicals, makeup, body lotions, nail polish, dental amalgam fillings, and root canals are some other toxic products many of us use every day that are loaded with chemicals and substances that are foreign to our bodies.

Fluoride

Did you know that fluoride is a toxic industrial by-product that is captured in the scrubber system from the manufacturing process of phosphate fertilizer products and as such is a poison? It may also contain lead, mercury, arsenic, and cadmium. Manufacturers sell this toxic by-product to municipalities instead of paying to have it disposed of in a toxic waste dump facility. The municipalities then use it to fluoridate our drinking water.

Fluoride is rejected by most of the rest of the industrialized world because they have elected politicians who care about the health of those countries' residents. Check the warning label on your tube of toothpaste. Fluoride can cause death from overdose. How safe can it really be if the label warns of calling the poison control center if accidentally swallowed? It's not only used in just toothpaste anymore, it's also an ingredient in many popular mouthwashes. Massive amounts of fluoridated water may also be used by processed food manufacturers, so trace amounts fluoride may be present in those foods as well.

Dental Fluorosis, Skeletal Fluorosis, and Fluoroderma

Fluoride can also cause mottled brown teeth in children who consume water high in fluoride. This condition is known as dental fluorosis. How do you know if your child will be affected? You don't know. How much is too much is relative to each child's capacity to filter out the fluoride. Research has also shown a relationship between fluoride consumption and brittle bones, a condition now known as skeletal fluorosis. Fluoride can also cause an acute cystic acne condition known as fluoroderma.

So, tell me again, why is fluoride in our water supply? Why is anything in our water supply that doesn't belong there? Why do we consciously add toxic substances? (Mercola.com "Warning Never Swallow Regular Toothpaste" 2013).

Fluoride and Fluoroderma

One woman, named Melissa (no last name given), experienced a really profound case of acne, with cystic outbreaks that started while she was in her teens and continued right through college and into adulthood. She tried all the usual forms of prescription drugs and over the counter drug treatments, but nothing would eliminate it. As a student she took trips to study abroad in Europe and Africa and discovered while in those countries her acne either considerably lessened or vanished. Oddly, when she returned to the United States, her acne reappeared. After repeated attempts at trying to resolve this with drug therapy, she became frustrated and decided she wanted to get to the cause of her acne, not just treat the symptoms. Not only did she find her acne was caused by a severe sensitivity to fluoride in her diet (it's not just in the water), but she went through a very uncomfortable and sometimes painful detoxification process. Melissa documented all she went through, including the detoxification process, and wanted to share her experience, so she wrote a seventy-four page e-book called *Healing Acne from Within—How to Diagnose and Cure Acne Caused by Fluoride Exposure*. There are eleven pages of references at the end of the book. Melissa really did her homework. The book is a free download or you can view it online on her website. Melissa started this website because she was initially interested in exploring how to eliminate cellulite, and the website now includes her fluoride story and related research as well. (Cellulite Investigation 2011)

Other sources of fluoride can also be found in wine, beer, tea, soda, chicken, fish whose bones are eaten (like anchovies and sardines), cereals, and vegetables. Here are a couple of reasons. One, the food may be grown and processed using fluoridated water. Two, the feed given to animals grown in controlled farming, like chicken and cattle farming, is grown using fluoridated water.

If you have a high sensitivity to fluoride it's best to use as much organically grown fruits and vegetables as possible. If you eat animal protein, look for fish that's caught wild, and for chicken and beef, make sure it's free-range and pasture-raised.

Water-Quality Report—a Municipality in Florida

Here is part of a water-quality report from a town in Florida, which clearly shows fluoride is in the municipal water supply there, the parts per million, and the likely source of the contamination. If the community you live in fluoridates the water, you should be able to obtain a water-quality report from them. They may even be required to send you one periodically if you're a homeowner in the community.

Contaminant and Unit of Measurement—Fluoride (ppm)

Date sample taken (MO/YR)	03/11
MCL Violation Y/N	N
Level Detected	0.12 PPM
Range of Results	N/A
MCLG	4
MCL	4.0
Likely Source of Contamination	Erosion of natural deposits; discharge from fertilizer and aluminum factories; water additive which promotes strong teeth when at optimum levels between 0.7 and 1.3 PPM

The important thing here is the likely source of contamination and the justification they use for including it: "promotes strong teeth when at optimum levels ..." If you read Melissa's online, seventy-four page e-book about the history of fluoride and the clearly summarized research, you'll quickly understand how and why fluoride came into use. I still contend that fluoride, among other contaminants, does not belong in our water supply. If it's in our water, it's in everything else we consume, too.

You can find even more information about the dangers of fluoride at the Fluoride Action Network. (fluoridealert.org "Frequently Asked Questions" 2012)

Where Does the Fluoride Added to Water Come From?

The main fluoride chemical added to water (hydrofluorosilicic acid) is an industrial by-product of the phosphate fertilizer industry. Unlike the fluoride used in toothpaste, hydrofluorosilicic acid is not pharmaceutical-grade quality. It is an unpurified, industrial-grade, corrosive acid that has been linked, in several recent studies, to increased levels of lead in children's blood.

I could not find any reports on how the pharmaceutical-grade quality fluoride is different from the hydrofluorosilicic acid or why pharmaceutical-grade quality fluoride would be any better for adding to toothpaste than hydrofluorosilicic acid.

What Are Potential Risks from Consuming Fluoridated Water?

Health risks associated with low-to-moderate doses of fluoride include dental fluorosis, bone fracture, bone cancer, joint pain, skin rash, reduced thyroid activity, and IQ deficits.

Is Fluoridated Water Safe for Babies?

No. Although The American Dental Association (ADA) has since retracted this recommendation, they initially suggested that children under one year of age should not receive infant formula made with fluoridated water.

However, other research studies support this initial recommendation. Fluoride can pass over the blood brain barrier of a developing fetus and can contribute to a child developing dental fluorosis—a tooth defect caused by fluoride-induced cell damage within the teeth, among developing other side effects in the longer term. Chemicals that find their way into a baby's bloodstream can penetrate into the brain. (fluoridealert.org "Brain" 2012)

My Comment

So, again, why is something as potent as fluoride restricted from babies up to one year old and then, magically, when they turn one year old, they suddenly become immune to it, or are able to better tolerate it? Suddenly, when babies turn one year old, their livers are able to process the fluoride out? What about the rest of their lives and into adulthood? This does not make any sense to me. There are multiple studies that show this, yet fluoride is still allowed in our water supplies. Is it any wonder we have chronic disease problems here in America?

Worse than the dental fluorosis is the suggestion that fluoride can interfere with brain function. Thirty-six studies completed, as of September 2012, investigated the relationship between fluoride and human intelligence and they showed that "elevated fluoride exposure is associated with reduced IQ…" (fluoridealert.org "Fluoride & Intelligence: The 36 Studies" 2012)

There is so much information about the perils of fluoride that I am appalled at why it is still an added ingredient to so many oral products and our water supply. So again I ask, why?

Laundry Detergents, Fabric Softeners, and Cleaning Products

All of these products contain harmful chemicals that don't belong in our storehouse of cleaning products for laundry or windows, or on our bodies as a result of using them. There are much safer alternative options available.

Makeup, Body Lotions, Nail Polish, and Nail Polish Remover

Spend some time looking at the ingredient list in these products. You may choose to never bring them in your house again or get a manicure or pedicure using nail polish and nail polish remover. Makeup and body lotions, especially sun-tan lotion, really clog your pores and prevent your skin from breathing. Nadine Artemis has a wonderful line of skin care products that are all created using plant-based products that treat your skin with love and tenderness. (livinglibations 2012)

In Naples, Florida, there's a place called the Salt Cave, Inc. and a massage therapist named Erik who uses a cocoa butter mixture that he makes himself when giving the most incredible energy healing massage. That's about the extent I go into using products other than flax, coconut, avocado, and olive oils on my body. The Salt Cave is a very special spiritual and healing place. (Salt Cave 2012)

I use flax oil on my skin after I've been in the sun for a while, but I never use any sunscreen on my body unless it's from a source I know doesn't use chemical additives. Flax oil, believe it or not, is so good for your skin. I use it on my face and on any cuts I may get, and it helps to makes my skin soft and heals the cut at the same time.

The sun is good for you without suntan lotion. Just don't overdo it, especially if you don't live in an area where sun bathing is a daily habit for you. Dr. Joseph Mercola offers many healthier body products, so if you insist on using a sunscreen lotion or a skin-care product, please visit his website and explore some better options. (Mercola.com "Sunscreen & Tanning" 2013)

Dental Detoxing and Root Canals

Mercury exposure from mercury dental fillings, also known as *silver* fillings and *amalgams,* is a life-long threat. When a person chews, drinks, swallows, and breathes, mercury released from dental fillings is absorbed by the lungs and the linings of the digestive system into the bloodstream. As the fillings corrode, mercury fillings release ionized mercury into the saliva, tooth pulp, and gum tissues leading to the digestive system and bloodstream.

It's amazing to me that the amount of mercury used in just one filling is not allowed to be placed in a toxic waste dump. Mercury is a poison and has been used in "silver" amalgam fillings for years. Metal in your mouth also interrupts the body's natural energy flow, like a magnet. You can eliminate all metal in your mouth by going to a biological dentist who has had special training in the proper removal of amalgam fillings and replacement with a composite filling that will not cause a disruption in your body's energy flow.

Root canals are a source of bacteria that can cause and create harmful effects in other areas of your body and organs. When a dentist performs a root canal, the tools used to clean out the pulp from the tooth cannot get into the microscopic channels in other parts of your tooth. These paths or grooves contain anaerobic bacteria. Anaerobic means bacteria can survive without oxygen. The bacteria continue to flourish and eliminate toxins from processing dead cells. The surrounding blood supply and lymph system allow the toxins to spread to other areas of your body where they can set up shop in other organs and begin an infection, possibly creating a disease.

Dr. Mercola suggests the use of "non-reactive metal implants made from zirconium." Non-reactive means that you body might not react adversely to a foreign substance.

(Mercola.com "Why You Should Avoid Root Canals Like the Plague" 2013)

Marketing and Advertising

Why aren't humans at least as smart as our wonderful wild and not-so-wild kingdom friends? The answer is that we've been sold a lifetime of marketing crap on television, billboards, and radio, as well as in the super market, newspapers, and magazines. Now, with computer marketing, it's everywhere. It all started when you were a baby and your parents sat you in front of the TV for entertainment, or at least for me that's where it started.

Product information of every kind is drilled into you, just like you're in the military and your training instructor is in your face making sure you understand there is no deviation from his or her commands. I'm not saying every product is worthless; I'm saying you must practice discernment. Be skeptical; learn to listen, then go research the product. Look at the ingredient list, especially that of all processed food.

I was in a health-food store the other day and was tempted to buy "easy" bottled salad dressing. Well, sure enough, after reading the ingredient list, there it was: natural flavors added. You may think I'm overreacting on this natural-flavor concern; most of my friends think I'm nuts. However, Dr. Blaylock was very clear in his presentation about natural flavors and spices. Even some foods sold in health-food stores may not be the healthiest for you. You need to understand the ingredients contained in what you buy. I put the dressing down and left the store with my grocery cart full of produce and no packaged products. My better sense won over, and I made a real tasty dressing with lemon, lime, a bit of olive oil and a touch of raw honey. Yum!

Every product manufacturer has its own agenda, first and foremost. They are big business, in business to make money for their shareholders. The long-term outcome and effect on the health of people buying their products may not necessarily be the first thing they think about when they get up every morning. It should be, but it's not always the case.

You really need to remember that you still have choices. Food and product manufacturers are sparing no expense in creating new frozen, packaged, and boil-bag food items every day. They want you to buy and eat them, lots of them. They stress the convenience, the *easy* nature of their product. There's even milk in a box that needs no refrigeration. Yuck. I'm not saying marketing is bad; everyone has a right to make a living, but sometimes with the intensity of the advertising we become so drawn in as to become robotic. These marketing and advertising campaigns are powerful, and we subliminally succumb to the greatness of the product, buy, and become addicted to it.

For example, do you remember the little green gecko and the cave men who sell insurance? Those commercials were humorous, downright funny at times, and made a huge impression. Even if you didn't need the insurance right then and there, you were going to remember those characters and of course the insurance company when the time came to consider it. Everybody was talking about it.

Then there is the cute brunette all dressed in white with a brightly colored headband in a retail-sales showroom surrounded by tall, white, file-cabinet-like containers with different insurance product names on them. In walks a guy looking for insurance who works for another insurance company, and he's sheepishly caught by another co-worker also there doing the same thing. You're going to remember that one also.

Then there are the totally useless, in my opinion, ads for beauty products. How about that single-edge shaver that's coated with oil for women to use to make their legs look as sexy as the woman advertising it, who has long, dark, brown hair flowing down to the middle of her back with the gold dress on? Come on, folks! Can a shaver really make you look like that? No, of course it can't, and you know it. (Besides, the oil they put on those things just clogs up your pores anyway, and I wouldn't use one if you paid me.) Yet, when it comes time to buy your next shaver, I bet you're going to look at that one and consider it a possibility. Why, because this commercial made an immense impression on you.

The same is true of the processed-food industry. Just look at all the products being sold in the grocery store that have nothing to do with fresh fruits and vegetables. As far as I'm concerned, there are only two aisles necessary in any grocery store, one for produce and one for spices. The rest is just junk food, products that we don't need and that are only in those stores to help boost profit margins. Again, many of them are bought for convenience and ease of use.

The only difference in marketing between insurance and processed-food products is the processed food products are addictive. You can't eat and be addicted to insurance. But processed food, yes, a thousand times, yes.

We forget that we are human consumers and not robots. We can think for ourselves, and when presented with all the facts can make decisions for ourselves based on as much information as we can gather. The dollars the food manufacturers have to spend easily outweigh grass-roots groups and organic farmers who would like to promote their healthy options. The marketing ploys used by processed-food manufacturers define the speedy, easy, and healthy nature of using these products. They are manipulating the buying public into believing these products are healthy and OK for you to consume—right? Especially the easy part, we all like that in this busy day and age.

Take a look around at what's in some shopping carts the next time you go to the market and at the people pushing those carts. Are they filled with fresh fruits and vegetables and whole grain breads, or are they overflowing with microwave pizzas, microwavable single-serving dinners, toaster pastries, deli meats full of nitrites and nitrates, cheese, frozen waffles, soda, beer, wine, potato chips, and corn chips? Which family do you think is going to be consuming the highest amount of nutrition, and which one has been robotically reeled in disillusioned by the marketing?

Just take a look at the drug ads on TV. It seems anyone who may have a symptom close to what the drug is being marketed for suddenly is concerned about getting to the doctor. Gee, if I have this symptom and I can take a drug to relieve it, why not? In my opinion, the ad could actually create in some people a need for the drug, even if there isn't yet a symptom.

As you watch the man or woman smiling in the background, the narrator is talking about how great the drug is and how it can help you overcome your symptoms. Then, before the ad is over, you see a plethora of disclaimers about the horrible, potential, side effects of this drug, while the actors are still smiling and feeling oh so wonderful, totally ignoring the side effects being given to you, the viewer. When you see a drug ad in the newspaper or magazine, it's not an eighth of a page, a quarter page, a half page, or even a full page. It's usually three pages long. The first page spells out the drug, with pictures of happy, smiling, people, feeling great, for taking this drug. The next two pages are the disclaimers explaining the alarming side effects and the drug's contents listed in small print. Do you ever read the last two pages to see that this drug could actually cause death in certain circumstances? Who has that kind of money to spend on advertising? The drug companies do. That's why when it's time for the

Super Bowl some people tune in to watch, even if they couldn't care less about football. They want to watch the new ads for beer, cars, insurance products, wardrobe malfunctions, etc. Some of them are indeed quite clever. Kudos to the marketing professionals who think of ways to get and grab our attention; you are creative.

Beware and be aware of the claims made by these drugs and the double-blind studies that have been done regarding potent and potentially harmful pharmaceutical drugs. Do you know that there have been over *three-million deaths* caused by the side effects of prescription drugs that were dispensed and taken according to directions and zero deaths caused by nutritional supplements? (Natural News.com "Twenty-seven years brings no deaths from vitamins but over three million from pharmaceuticals" 2013)

Interesting isn't it? Something is dreadfully wrong and something is incredibly right with that picture. However, there is no big money to be made on nutritional supplements or organic fruits and vegetables because the drug companies can't patent natural substances.

The ads we view day in and day out, beginning when we were very little children watching cartoons on Saturday morning, make lasting impressions. Once the food manufacturers emotionally hook us into buying their products, they turn around and hook us physically, so much so that even today I occasionally have a *craving* for some Doritos. It's not really a craving, not now, as I'm pretty much toxin free and know that my grocery cart is filled with the fresh fruits and vegetables that will provide plenty of nutrition and antioxidants. The craving can be part of a lifelong pattern that was just simply an old habit, a habit that I was addicted to both emotionally and physically.

Ever wonder why you "can't eat just one?" Because, you can't. The MSG and other food additives described above cause us to be addicted. Old habits and lifestyle patterns die hard, and addicts of every kind have a tough time getting over their addiction. The memories of the smell, the taste, and the emotional circumstances surrounding old habits are incredibly ingrained in us. Even when we know how detrimental certain habits are, they can still take years to be fully released. That is, unless you're faced with a life-threatening health challenge or can get some psychological help to overcome the addiction. I know we've all heard it before, but it's true. We must become informed and educated consumers. I believe we put way too much trust in our government organizations and administrations that are supposed to be there to protect us but are not doing their job very well.

We also need to get back to the kitchen with the help of our families. Over the course of a lifetime, we've become creatures of excessive convenience, convicts of a chemically infused processed-food supply that's a far cry from real food. A few kitchen supplies and a couple of high-end small appliances like a Champion Juicer, Vitamix blender, and a wheatgrass juicer is all you need to outfit your kitchen for healthy raw food preparation. You don't even need to cook! How cool is that. I hope you're shopping at some farmers markets so you can save some money on produce and help out the local farming community as well.

We need to become informed consumers who can make educated decisions about what to put into our grocery carts so that what goes into our bodies is going to sustain them, not detain them.

Toxic Drugs

I no longer watch much television because the negative news is so overwhelming. If you believe everything everyone else is telling you, then you become a follower of someone else's prescription for life. "…almost half of the U.S. population is currently diagnosed with a chronic condition and 40 percent of people older than 60 are taking five or more medications." (Natural News.com "The racket that is Big Pharma" 2013)

Take this drug for this, take that drug for that. People over sixty are taking an average of five or more prescription medications each day? Come on, this is just outrageous and this is an average—some take more, and some take less. I don't believe this is a natural part of aging. I believe it's a side effect of a body deteriorated from a lifetime of consuming a diet of processed foods and living a toxic lifestyle of never-ending stress. If you think it's a natural part of aging, think again.

Prescription drug deaths increased 68 percent over a five-year period from 1999 to 2004 as Americans consumed yet more prescription drugs. "Poisoning from prescription drugs has risen to become the second-largest cause of unintentional deaths in the United States, according to the federal Centers for Disease Control and Prevention." (Natural News.com "Prescription drug deaths skyrocket 68 percent as Americans swallow more pills" 2013)

There are no known reported deaths from the consumption of any nutritional supplements. How toxic are prescription drugs to our bodies over our lifetime if the number of deaths attributed to them keeps rising? Prescription drugs combined with the Standard American Diet and a destructive lifestyle make a recipe for an early life departure. This surely makes no sense to me.

Alkalize Your Body

Our bodies need to be slightly more alkaline to maintain our health; disease cannot live in an alkaline environment. Disease likes the acid environment of our Standard American Diet, which is one reason we age faster than if we continuously ate and drank alkaline food and water.

The pH scale runs from 0-14, and we're born with a blood pH of around 7.365, which is about in the middle of the scale. If our blood pH varies too much from that, quite simply we can die. If your body isn't getting the alkalizing minerals it needs from the food and water you give it, your very intelligent body draws the alkalizing minerals it needs from inside. Your body wants to *live*! It will do everything it can to maintain that pH level, with or without your help, yet there are consequences.

Your body robs alkalizing minerals, calcium, phosphorous, and magnesium from your bones, teeth, and muscle tissue. So what happens then to your bones, teeth, and tissues when they are robbed of alkalizing minerals they need to keep them strong? They start to break down. You get osteoporosis, periodontal disease, and decreased muscle mass. And what happens to all that extra calcium and magnesium that is traveling throughout your bloodstream? Some of it is deposited into places it doesn't belong, wreaking havoc with those areas. These minerals get stuck in your joints, contributing to arthritis. Some of them get deposited onto your artery walls, contributing to clogged arteries and heart disease.

There is an answer. You can eat an alkalizing diet of primarily organic raw fruits and vegetables, drink alkaline water, and stop eating and drinking dead food and beverages in order to maintain the alkalinity needed to avoid the side effects mentioned above.

I recently did a simple at-home test with three different water samples. One sample was straight out of the cold water faucet. One sample was taken directly from my reverse osmosis water purification system. The third sample was water from my reverse osmosis system treated with a *pinch* of baking soda. Baking soda increases alkalinity, softens the water somewhat, and makes the water taste just a bit smoother. I purchased some pH test strips, which measure the pH level of liquids being tested. You can also use them to determine the pH of your urine and saliva. It was no surprise to me what the test strips showed:

Water right out of the tap measured a pH of 5.0

Water right out of the reverse osmosis system measured a pH of 4.5

Reverse osmosis with baking soda measured a pH of 7.0

You may wonder why the tap water measured 5.0 and the reverse osmosis measured 4.5. Tap water, in spite of the myriad of toxic chemicals, almost always measures higher on the pH scale than reverse osmosis because reverse osmosis water is so pure it's virtually devoid of any mineral content that could cause it to be anything but low on the pH scale. So believe it or not, the pinch of baking soda raised the pH level of the reverse osmosis water to a level almost equal to what our blood needs to keep our body healthy.

I had read about baking soda raising the pH level before but never tested it out. I realize this was a very crude at-home test, but it makes sense to me. So now I use a bit of baking soda in my water glass, knowing the alkalinity is closer to what my body needs to stay healthy. You could also add a squeeze of fresh lemon juice. The calcium and magnesium minerals from my bones, teeth, and muscles are going to stay where they belong—in my bones, teeth, and muscles. The economics of baking soda make it a simple solution to adding alkalizing water to your diet without having to spend a fortune. You can also take some baking soda with you when you travel so you can add it to your bottled water. You want to purchase aluminum-free baking soda.

You want to keep your body slightly alkaline, around 7.365. All cooked food and dairy products are acid forming. All raw foods are alkaline forming and disease cannot live in an alkaline environment.

Here's another experiment I did—this time on my body. I occasionally get a cold sore, usually in my nasal cavity. If you've ever had one you know it takes about ten days to disappear completely, no matter what you take or put on it. I tried all kinds of over-the-counter things years ago, and nothing ever seemed to help, except a prescription drug that when taken early enough did seem to arrest it. That was in the past, before I saw the errors of my old habits. I haven't taken any prescription drugs in over seven years.

If you're prone to cold sores, you know when you're getting one. You get that little itchy, tingling feeling, followed by blisters, followed by the soreness, scabbing, and finally the healing. We all know that these cold sores are actually an outbreak of a herpes virus that can lie dormant in your liver until you have a cause for these little buggers to parade around your face. So one day I got that *tingling feeling*. I thought, *Crap, I hate these things. What am I going to do?* If herpes is a virus, and a virus cannot live in an alkaline environment, and baking soda is alkaline, then guess what happened? I ran to the kitchen, opened up the kitchen cabinet, and pulled out the aluminum-free baking soda. This particular outbreak was inside my nose, so I took the baking soda, went to the bathroom, pulled out a cotton swab, wet the swab and dipped it into the baking soda. Then I managed to coat the inside of my nose where the cold sore was with the baking soda. I did this first thing in the morning, immediately after I woke up, when I discovered the cold sore coming on.

I went about my morning, and when it came time for a shower, I went to wash my face with flax oil and discovered my cold sore no longer itched or tingled and appeared to be significantly improved over what it felt like when I woke up just a few hours earlier. By the end of the day, the cold sore no longer bothered me. If I pressed on the outside of my nose, I could tell something was still there, but nothing like what it would have been if it had gone untreated. I was fairly symptom-free in less than twenty-four hours using plain old baking soda!

I was dancing with a friend a few weeks ago, and several of us were gathered around a table talking. One friend mentioned that she just got over a very unsightly cold sore on her upper lip, just under her nostrils. You could still see the scarred and darkened area. The other friend, who was a nurse, mentioned the prescription drug I used to take years ago, and the friend with the cold sore feverishly wrote down the name of the drug so she could get some from her doctor in the event of a future outbreak. I mentioned my recent experience with the baking soda to her.

The nurse friend said, "Oh, that's an old fashioned remedy."

"So what?" I said to myself. Let me see, put unknown chemicals into my body or plain old aluminum-free baking soda. Gee, to me that's a no-brainer, but I'm already on the other side, the side of "First do no harm."

The nurse friend had an *attitude* about my suggesting the aluminum-free baking soda; I knew she hailed from the camp of Western medicine. The look was on her face. She knew best because she's in the medical profession and knows these things. I know she was trying to help. However, when she admitted knowing about the baking soda remedy and continued to suggest a prescription drug, it just did not compute. You know that old acronym KISS? Keep It Simple Stupid. Why complicate things? Let me see, call your doctor, hope you get through on the first call, probably at least a ten-dollar co-pay, drive to and from the drug store, and end up taking a toxic drug. Compare that to aluminum-free baking soda, which is probably in your kitchen cupboard, just over three dollars on the Vitacost website, no co-pay, no travel time, no inconvenience.

It amazes me to see so many people lost in the world of prescription drugs. I read testimonials on the Internet and hear testimonials from personal acquaintances who are normal, everyday, run-of-the-mill folks who cured their diseases and illnesses. They did this using juicing, raw food, detoxing, and creating a healthy lifestyle. Yes, of course, medical doctors are necessary for diagnostic, emergency, and many other essential medical services. I welcome them in those times and places, and so will you. But I'm here to help you understand that healing your body from diseases related to unhealthy lifestyle excesses does not have to be painful, convoluted, or difficult.

Dairy Products

Actually, milk and other dairy products weaken the bones and accelerate osteoporosis. That's right, consumption of milk causes the very condition it's advertised to prevent.

As I'll explain in the next story, osteoporosis results from calcium loss, not necessarily insufficient calcium intake. And dairy products, because of their high protein content, promote calcium loss. Studies examining the incidence of osteoporosis have found that high consumption of dairy products is associated with high rates of osteoporosis. If you want strong bones, don't drink milk. (Borio Chiropractic Health Center "Dairy – Milk, is "Udder" Nonsense" 2013)

Dairy products are a key cause of constipation. They contain casein, a protein that the human body isn't designed to digest. It goes into the bowel undigested, leading to a general *gumming up* of the system. This is true in both adults and in young people. If your intestinal track is all gummed up, how can any other nutrients get through their walls to sustain you? They can't.

Dr. John A. McDougall, a physician and nutrition expert, says that dairy products are strongly linked as a potential cause in a variety of illnesses, especially allergies. Cow's milk and products made from cow's milk contain proteins that can induce adverse reactions in our bodies.

We are the only animal on the planet that drinks the milk of another animal. Our bodies and immune system were meant to drink mother's milk as babies and after that, pure water and juices. Our body's immune system has no idea what to do with proteins that aren't part of our makeup. When that happens, sometimes it begins an attack in response that could be the basis or cause of a host of other autoimmune diseases.

Some conditions that could be caused by or linked to dairy products are loss of appetite, growth retardation, upper gastrointestinal disorders, lower gastrointestinal disorders, respiratory ailments, skin conditions, bone-and-joint problems, nervous-system issues related to behavior, and blood disorders.

Give up the dairy, not for the hell of it, but for the health of it!

Oxygenate Your Body

You need air to breathe, and your cells need oxygen to function properly. You are made up of approximately seventy trillion cells, and what do you think causes you to breathe? The efficient functioning of every living and breathing *cell* in each and every organ and system in your body. Your cells are you. Each cell, as microscopic as it is, has an independent operating system, just like your body as a whole. It needs to take in nourishment, to breathe, to exhale, and to eliminate waste products.

People think, *Sure, I'm breathing.* But there is a difference between breathing and really breathing to live. That is why a lot of hospitalized patients are given oxygen, to help support their breathing and recovery.

Everyone needs to get some exercise each day in order to keep the body oxygenated. Walk, ride your bike, take the stairs instead of the elevator, jump on a mini trampoline. The mini trampoline, also called a rebounder, can give you an hour's worth of exercise in just fifteen minutes, and it's easy on your joints, comes with a handle bar, and is compact and easy to store. I use mine in front of the television as I watch HGTV. That's about the only show I do watch. Fifteen minutes go by in no time, and I feel refreshed and ready to go take on the day. Sometimes I pick up some light, one-to-three- pound weights and exercise my arms at the same time. You can get a rebounder for around $100.

Another easy-to-use piece of exercise equipment is called a whole-body vibration machine. Ten minutes on one of these and you've again done about an hour of regular exercise at the gym. In both cases you've exercised your whole body, shaken loose some toxins from your lymph system, and most importantly brought some badly needed oxygen to your cells. The whole-body vibration system is also very easy on the joints. All you do with this equipment is stand there, and the machine does the rest. How cool is that? This equipment is a bit more expensive, though. Check them out.

In both of the above cases there are no monthly gym fees, no transportation needed, just the desire and will to use the equipment at home. If you walk regularly there is no cost of equipment and plenty of fresh air.

Eating a diet high in fats and white carbohydrates makes it difficult for your blood to carry oxygen easily and efficiently throughout your body. Eating organic fresh fruits and vegetables allows your blood to carry nutrients and oxygen throughout all parts of your body with ease.

Think of a kitchen strainer, the kind you use for straining pasta or sifting flour. See how easily the water pours through the strainer? That's what your intestines go through to deliver nutrients and oxygen to your entire body. If you had a pound of fat or butter in that strainer, not much would get though, right? So eating a diet high in organic fruits and vegetables will be a sure-fire way to get the nutrients you need into the areas of your body that need them.

Chapter Summary

When I was in Colorado Springs at HealthQuarters and heard about this information for the first time, it shocked me to learn that many of the processed-food products sold as food in the United States that I was consuming were just plain toxic.

We truly need to keep an open mind about all of these things and do the best we can in making our decisions. As I stated at the beginning of this book, my goal and purpose in this effort is make you aware of the many nontoxic solutions and choices available as you journey into a healthier you. HealthQuarters Ministries made me aware, and I want to pay this tribute forward so you don't have to go through breast cancer or other diseases. You can avert a serious illness and teach your children and grandchildren about the life-giving and sustaining value of pure organic fruits and vegetables and how to live long and prosper.

Your heart is in your hands, no one else's. Enjoy your responsibility, own it. You have the power; you can make decisions for yourself. This is freedom; this is fabulous!

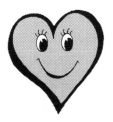

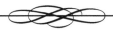

CHAPTER 6

Dead Food Funeral and the Clean Out

MY LIFE CHANGED THE INSTANT I heard I had breast cancer. The exhausting hours of research, an eight-day stay at HealthQuarters, and all the information I learned there caused me to reflect on what my diet and lifestyle were like up to that point. All I knew was that I was not going to give up; neither did I expect or want to die.

Just about everything I learned about diet and lifestyle growing up needed to be trashed. I'm not criticizing my mother, father, or other family members for giving me a lot of bad information. They were just giving me what they knew to be true based on their own set of values passed on from their parents, one generation to the next.

My life, my health, my diet, my entire body changed overnight. It is one of the best things that's ever happened to me. This change became my purpose in life. I became alive and vibrant with a renewed determination—to apply all that I learned, cure my disease called cancer, and share my story.

I came home from HealthQuarters and went through everything in my house, not just the food in the refrigerator. I was a white tornado!

Refrigerator

When I learned about all the chemical additives that are put into our food, I started reading labels seriously, with intention, especially the ones on prepared food in cans, jars, and bottles in my refrigerator and freezer.

Bill occasionally would ask me if something in the fridge was OK to eat, knowing it had been there for a while. I would tease him and say, that stuff has so many preservatives in it I'm sure it's OK, especially since it wasn't turning brown or growing any green fuzzy stuff like mold. Boy was I right, but I didn't know just how right I was. Neither did I know the consequences of what these chemical preservatives could do to our bodies and ultimately our health over the long term. I have had a few forgotten foreigners in the fridge that became penicillin experiments after a few months, but at least those actually made it into the trash!

Needless to say, most of the *food* in the refrigerator was replaced with a fresher, organic, nontoxic counterpart, especially when it came to the condiments like mayonnaise, ketchup, pickles, jellies, jams, peanut butter, milk, and cheeses. Take ketchup for example. There's a lot of information out there on the pitfalls of high-fructose corn syrup. The major food manufacturers are now coming up with their own organic high-fructose corn syrup-free versions of many condiments. Annie's was the only nontoxic, high-fructose corn syrup-free option available that I knew of in 2005, so that's the one I chose. I used to lather up my burgers, french fries, and just about any other kind of meat with a thick layer, edge to edge, of toxic ketchup. The ketchup wasn't just on the burger, but I had to dip the burger into a side of ketchup in addition to the slather already on the bun. I might as well have eaten a ketchup sandwich. *Ugh!*

Regular mayonnaise was another one that was tough to give up. I would spread it on a both slices of bread, also edge-to-edge. I think it was my addiction to the condiment that made the sandwich so good, not the meat, cheese, tomato, and lettuce. The mayo had to be thick, plentiful, and easy to slide down my throat.

I truly believe part of the ketchup and mayo habit was the addictive nature of the additives. And high-fructose corn syrup is also very addictive. It was a difficult chore to give up these things, but my mind was made up. If I was going to follow this program, I was going in all the way!

I no longer eat ketchup of any kind, except on very rare occasions (I do indulge ever so infrequently in some sweet potato fries), so I really didn't mind giving up the slathering activities. I had two other burger and fry eaters in the house, so I couldn't eliminate it from everyone's diet even though I wanted to. I was an outlaw as it was, straying away from the med school graduates, their wisdom, and acumen. My family wasn't keen on this idea at all, but this was my journey, not theirs. I needed to feel empowered, and HealthQuarters gave me all the empowerment I needed.

Spice Cabinet

Be truthful now, how many of you received a spice rack or even two for a shower or wedding gift decades ago? Do you still have some of those spices and dried herbs lingering, now gaunt and gray, in the back corner of your spice shelf, dead and lifeless? If you didn't notice, my hand went up! I couldn't believe it when I took one of those pitiful jars, unscrewed the top, and smelled the contents. What smell? They were so dried out that even under cover for years they were nearly scentless and indescribable. Things do go bad after a while, even if they are dried and covered in an airtight container. Where did that smell go? Come on now, these can't be good for you, let alone do anything to enhance the flavor of the rare recipe you might make when those spices and herbs are required.

Throw out the spice or herb contents but save the glass jars for future smaller purchases of frequently used dried herbs and spices and label them yourself. It's best to get these from a health-food store that sells the organic version. When the need comes to use a rare dried spice or herb that you don't regularly store, buy it when you need it; your taste buds will thank you. Better yet, buy fresh herbs and spices; all of them have health benefits. It takes double the amount of fresh herbs to equal an amount of dry herbs to flavor any recipe.

Whew! That was a tough job. I think I had a whole cabinet of shelf space available after that exercise. Don't be so frugal you can't throw things out. We're talking about your life here.

The Can Pantry

This was the toughest job, getting rid of the accumulation of canned goods—you know, the just-in-case-you-need-something-in-a-hurry kind of food. How convenient is a carrot or a celery stick for quick food? Now I know. Bill still had some rations from when he served in the National Guard, all in dark-green, military, colored cans. Canned goods do last quite a long time past the expiration date, but that doesn't mean they're void of the toxic suspects that help the manufacturers add volume to their products and allow them to cost less. I threw out a ton of canned goods. And please don't feel inclined to feed these canned chemicals to the local food pantry, especially if the products have long since passed their expiration date. No science experiments in the can pantry, just old, lifeless canned goods.

Canned and bottled food items need to be brought to a temperature around 240 degrees F. to kill any bacteria to prolong the product's shelf life. Where's the food life? Where's the nutrient density? Where are the enzymes?

Now go have a dead-food funeral!

Under the Kitchen and Bathroom Sinks

Wow! Learning about toxic chemicals at HealthQuarters was a real eye opener. Our skin is the biggest organ in our body, well, really, *on* our body, but it is an organ. Our skin can absorb toxic chemicals though our pores, toxic sun-tan lotions, makeup, body and hand lotions, and just about anything else that we put on our skin.

OK. Here's another funny question. How many of you clean the shower and tub areas when you're naked, before you take your real shower? How many of you use powdered cleansers, and how many of you use those spray-on bath/tub/shower cleaners, *without using a pair of gloves*? I'm guilty as charged, or I used to be. It's always so much easier to really get things clean when you can go into full face-to-face combat with the dirt using cleansers, an old toothbrush, toothpicks, and cotton swabs when you don't have to worry about getting your clothes wet and soggy. When everything is clean, then you take a shower. Ahhhh, feels so good!

Just about all of these cleansers come with some kind of warning label on them. If they're inhaled, accidentally swallowed, get in your eyes, or come in contact with your skin they tell you to call the poison control center, call the doctor, and bring the container with you when you go to the hospital emergency room. "Keep out of reach of children and pets. Caution: Moderate eye and skin irritant. May be harmful if swallowed or inhaled. Read cautions on back." Holy Cow, Batman! These are some of the warnings on the can from just one type of common, everyday powdered cleanser.

The solution is aluminum-free baking soda and water or white vinegar and water. These two products can clean just about anything, and baking soda actually kills germs— in your mouth, in your kitchen sink, in your toilet bowl, everywhere. It's an alkaline substance, and germs can't live in an alkaline environment. Neither can disease live in a body that's alkaline. Baking soda also makes your skin soft, so use it in a warm bath and see how soft your skin feels after a twenty-minute soak. It's better than a bubble bath, and there's no toxicity.

We've been sold an incredible bill of goods because product manufacturers are competing with one another trying to make the next generation of best-ever-cleaning products that cut through hard-water build up, scale, and scum without scrubbing. Hogwash! I don't think I've used any of those products that didn't actually require a good old-fashioned scrubbing, even with all their claims. It seems the more improved a product gets, the harsher the chemicals.

I think we've all just become very lazy about cleaning. It seems to be regarded as something beneath us, and we'd rather have a cleaning service. It's exercise. Do it yourself; don't hire a cleaning service. Get down and get dirty with some environmentally safe cleaning products and wear some gloves. Put the bathroom fan on when you're cleaning in small spaces or open a window. Put on some fun, up-beat music to listen to as you clean.

Even Jesus cleaned his own room growing up! I don't know, just kidding!
Jesus was, however, a very humble being, and it wouldn't surprise me to
learn that he did.

Beauty Products

At HealthQuarters we learned about the chemical ingredients of makeup,
lotions, and colognes. My eyes grew even wider. Who could possibly
believe there are so many poisons in the composition of beauty products?
The words "poison" and "beauty" in the same sentence made me think of
David and Goliath or Beauty and the Beast. Poisonous beauty products—
how could this be? After all, the advertisements on television and in beauty
magazines show gorgeous women using these products, and these pictures
are meant to hook us. Just as I mentioned before with the ads for drugs,
these ads are intended to solicit us. Who wouldn't want to look and smell
like these dazzling women?

Mineral oil, alpha-hydroxy acids, formalin (which is actually
formaldehyde, used to preserve dead bodies), lacquer, and sodium lauryl
sulphate are just some toxic beauty product ingredients that harm your skin
in one way or another. They clog your pores and dry out your skin, causing
you to use more of the product. They can be skin irritants and cause skin
or other related allergies and make your skin more susceptible to harmful
UV rays from the sun. So where's the benefit? It's easy to believe a TV
commercial or a magazine ad. They're larger than life, right there in front
of you, begging you to purchase these products so you can look just like
these beautiful models. Chances are you're more like me—just a plain
Jane who loves who she is with all her flaws, nicks, and scars. My skin
is glowing because of the diet I eat, not because of any beauty products I
buy.

You want to believe what the ads say, right? The women using and
wearing these products cause you to believe they've used, worn, and been
buying these products for years and that these creams and moisturizers have
kept their skin looking young, smooth, and soft. These are just one-time
photos or advertisements that have been airbrushed and PhotoShopped to

death. We know this, yet we, as primarily female purchasers, keep buying cauldrons of toxic chemical creams, lotions, foundations, lipsticks, eye shadows, and mascara in the name of beauty.

We all have a natural beauty, and it comes out when we shine with our heart and soul, not just through the layers of beauty products we apply to our skin. Raw fruits and vegetables will go a longer way toward correcting and restoring beautiful skin than any dollar amount spent on beauty products. This food costs much less than these products, and you have to buy food anyway. Raw organic fruits and vegetables are all you need to correct any skin condition and eliminate disease.

Try making a mixture of one tablespoon each of avocado, coconut, and flax oils, then apply to your face and everywhere else on your body that needs moisturizing. I often add some essential oils; however, some essential oils can be very concentrated and harmful to your skin if not used properly. This mixture is quite economical and needs to be kept in the refrigerator because flax oil can spoil at room temperature. The coconut oil will cause the mixture to harden under the cooler temperature, but it's fine to use that way. Just dip your fingers in and gently apply on your face and any other part of your skin that needs moisturizing. These oils are food and not only soften your skin but are good for you. Please remember to use raw organic oils. I've experimented using just flax oil, and I like that, too. It's great to apply before and after going to the beach. Keeps dried skin nice and soft and supple. If you want to try this, please purchase a book on essential oils and do some research on which oils can be used on your skin. If that idea seems too complex, once again go to livinglibations and review Nadine Artemis's product line. It was in viewing her videos that I was inspired to make my own version of her products. Of course making your own is much more cost effective. Artemis shares information about the ancient Gypsy tradition of using pure and essential oils for cleansing and exfoliating your skin. Can you believe it, just pure oil, no chemical ingredients? Again, this makes perfect sense to me. Our skin is not made of chemicals. (livinglibations 2012)

This has been said a million times but needs repeating. Read the ingredient list; whether it's on food, makeup, or other products. If you can't pronounce an ingredient, it's probably some sort of chemical, and why on earth would you want to eat it, drink it, or put it on your body? What goes on your skin gets absorbed into your body.

Colognes and Perfumes

Ethyl alcohol, phthalates, and glycerin are common additives in making perfumes and are used primarily to extend the shelf life of the product. Extend the shelf life. Hmmm. Again, anything that needs life extending by chemical means just can't be good for you. Not to mention the smell of most of these products is just awful. There is nothing that turns me off more than smelling cologne on a man or woman, especially if it's overpowering. It quite literally makes me nauseous. How does a man or woman figure out chemistry in the opposite sex when it's all covered up with artificial scents? I want to smell the real thing. Ok, just me!

Here is the ingredient list from the label of a natural, organic, scented spray: "Filtered water, naturally brewed herbal vodka tincture, organic olive oil, organic lavender, organic bilberry leaf, absolute rose, organic geranium rose, absolute jasmine, organic ylang ylang, and organic sandalwood. This is packaged in a bio-energy glass. All natural, handmade, vegetarian, chemical-and-cruelty-free, never tested on animals, and organic as possible."

Now here's an excerpt from an article that appeared on the *Natural News* website from December 6, 2010 about the ingredient labeling requirements for cosmetic and personal care product manufacturers: "The Federal Fair Packaging and Labeling Act of 1973 explicitly exempts manufacturers of cosmetics and personal care products from having to disclose any of the ingredients used to give fragrance to their products, as long as 'fragrance' is listed on the label. This lack of disclosure becomes particularly dangerous when combined with a large-scale lack of data on the safety of these compounds; neither the FDA nor any publicly accountable organization has ever tested the majority of fragrance compounds for safety as ingredients in personal care products." (Natural News.com "Celebrity-branded perfumes loaded with toxic petrochemicals" 2013)

Which fragrance would you like to have on your body? A product whose ingredients are completely disclosed on the label and are part of the food chain, or one where the ingredients are hidden, untested, and exempt from any labeling at all, except listing the word *fragrance* on it?

It's just criminal that manufacturers of all kinds of products get away with nondisclosure in this country under congressionally passed laws. Who are we protecting and why? What's so *fair* about "The Federal Fair Packaging and Labeling Act of 1973"? You decide.

Laundry Room

Detergents, fabric softeners, spot removers, and bleach—Oh my! All contain similar chemicals and compounds that defy the imagination unless you're a research scientist who plays in that arena. The majority of us use these products to get the cleanest, whitest wash on the block. Gee, what would happen if we didn't add fabric softener to the wash or throw that drier sheet in the drier with the load of freshly-washed clothes? It would smell like freshly dried clothes, right? What's wrong with that? Why does it have to smell like anything other than what it is?

Clothing and Footwear

Believe it or not, many articles of clothing and shoes are made from a host of artificial fibers that can wear off and be absorbed into your skin. Our feet have the largest pores on our body, so be careful what kind of shoes, flip flops, or sandals you're wearing. It's unbelievable that so much footwear is made of rubber and plastic that it's darn near impossible to find a good shoe or sandal with an insole made of leather or suede, let alone an actual sole made of leather.

Rubber and plastic shoes are cheap to produce, market, and sell, and they can be made in all kinds of pretty bright colors. You never stop to think what the direct rubber or plastic contact with your skin may be doing to compromise your health. There are also many fabrics and shoes made from petroleum-based products. Over time, the molecules wear off the fabric or shoes, are absorbed through the pores, and travel into the bloodstream. We become sitting ducks and science experiments. We just don't know the consequences of how our body is going to handle these foreign invaders (called xenoestrogens, or fake estrogen) that mimic our natural estrogen.

When these fibers go into the body through the pores as microscopic particles and travel around the bloodstream, what happens? They wreak havoc with the body's ability to identify these foreign invaders and the body does not know what to do with them. Do they become part of your liver, heart, kidney, or pancreas? Do they lodge in your brain, become stuck in an artery wall, all of the above? Here are just a few familiar fabric names and their associated definitions from an on-line source.

What is Polyester?

"Polyester consists of 'long-chain polymers' that are derived from a chemical reaction involving coal, petroleum, air, and water. Specifically, a reaction between the petroleum by-products *alcohol* and *carboxyl acid* forms a compound that is known as a monomer or 'ester.' This reaction, which takes place at high temperatures, in a vacuum, is referred to as polymerization." (eHow.com "What Is Polyester Fabric Made From" 2013)

What Is Fleece?

"Utilizing advanced technology, polyester fibers are created from *terephthalic acid* and *ethylene glycol* (both made from petroleum) or from recycled plastic soda bottles. The fibers are twisted into yarn, which is woven or knit into fabric. The surface of the fabric is then brushed with wire brushes before it is trimmed (or sheared) to the desired length and finished." (eHow.com "What Is Fleece Fabric Made From" 2013)

What Is Spandex and Lycra?

These fabrics are similar in that they're both made from polymers, plastic, and oil. Do you really want these fibers on your skin all day long? These fabrics are manufactured using oil, acids, and coal. When your body sees foreign molecules, it doesn't know how to process them. It can't metabolize these foreign invaders, so these molecules get stuck somewhere in the body or bloodstream and can be the beginning of a real health problem. All of these products are filled with toxic chemicals, and many of these toxic elements aren't even listed on the labels of the products being sold.

Eco-friendly natural fibers are grown and produced without the use of any artificial fertilizers, pesticides, or chemicals. Natural fibers like cotton, wool, bamboo, linen, and silk are some of the naturally produced materials used to manufacture all kinds of products. Many natural fibers are spun to make wonderful clothing, sheets, towels, and pillows, and these fibers are sustainable and renewable and don't contain oil, coal, or acid.

What Are Xenoestrogens?

"Xenoestrogens are foreign estrogens. They are estrogen mimickers that affect the estrogen in our bodies and can alter hormone activity. Growing evidence implicates xenoestrogens in a wide range of human and wildlife health problems.

There are some 70,000 registered chemicals having hormonal effects, in addition to being toxic and carcinogenic. The synergistic effects of exposure are well documented, but largely unknown. These substances can increase the estrogen load in the body over time and are difficult to detoxify through the liver.

It is now being discovered that these synthetic estrogens are making their way into our bodies and pretending to be our biological estrogen. They are present in our soil, water, air, food supply, and personal care and household products." (Suite101 "Xenoestrogens and Your Health" 2013)

You have to remember that most of us spend around 40–50 percent of our lives in our homes—sleeping, cooking, reading, watching TV, playing games with our children, and entertaining our friends. The closer we can come to using truly natural products in and on our bodies and in our homes, the closer we can get to obtaining and maintaining a balanced state of health.

So many things, like the air we breathe and water we drink, are out of our control that we need to exercise control over the things we can so we reduce our overall exposure to toxic elements whose side effects even the experts aren't sure about.

The other 50–60 percent of the time we're in our cars, at work, out shopping, on vacations, or otherwise out of our home, and those are places we cannot control, so it's important to make our home environment as healthy and safe as possible.

Please remember that I'm someone who needed a total turnaround in my health. I employed as many toxin-reducing strategies that I could find. I was trying to recover from breast cancer. I wanted to live, so I persevered and changed my diet and lifestyle and subsequently changed my life. Reducing or eliminating every toxic exposure I could was critical to becoming whole again.

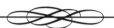

CHAPTER 7

Tools To Physically Detox Your Body

THE TOOLS FOR PHYSICAL DETOXING are gentle, yet unfamiliar. Please pay particular attention to this information so you can take a milder approach to cleaning up your systems before they really get out of whack and you're diagnosed with cancer, high blood pressure, heart disease, high cholesterol, diabetes, or other diseases. *All diseases result from a failed immune system*, which you and only you have control over.

Once you have a disease, the following methods may seem more extreme, compared to just taking a pill, but they work. However, if you're not already diagnosed with some brand of disease, then you can take steps like changing your diet and lifestyle to ward off any kind of alternative or conventional medical intervention.

What is Detoxing?

Simply put, detoxification is an intensified waste-management elimination system for your body. The purpose of detoxification is to assist the body in a clean-out process, which can take many different forms. Some or all of them can be applied at the same time or at different times, depending on your overall state of health and hopefully under the care of an alternative health care professional.

Juicing—Fresh Fruits and Vegetables

What is juicing exactly? It's using fresh fruits and vegetables with as much of the whole fruit as possible, including the skins and seeds, where possible, and passing them through some type of press or masticator, known as a juicer. Many people think of a juicer as a citrus juicer, where you cut the citrus in half and then rotate the fruit on the top of a spiral-type plastic or glass piece that extracts the juice. This is fine for fresh citrus juices, but it lacks the most important part of why you juice, which is to extract not just the juice from the pulp but to break down the fibers from the membranes in the fruit, seeds, and skins to draw out the enzymes.

Enzymes are the key reason you juice. Enzymes are the healing elements that will reinvent, rejuvenate, and restore your immune system. You can't live without enzymes, and I've devoted a whole chapter to them later on, so I won't get into them too deeply here except to say again, you can't live without them. It's really that simple. Your body is like a finely-woven piece of lace, with each strand of silk or yarn connecting ever so intricately to the next. Everything has to work together to keep you healthy, and when one part is missing, your body tries like hell to make up in other areas for what's lacking. But there are only so many places your intelligent body can go before it starts to give up and dry up. This is part of why we age.

Wheatgrass juice is the fountain of youth, the elixir of life. The similarities between wheatgrass juice and our own blood are almost identical. Dr. Jeffrey Dach says: "The intense green color of wheatgrass juice is due to the chlorophyll content. The molecular structure of chlorophyll is virtually identical to hemoglobin, the oxygen carrying red pigment of our blood." The main difference is that the nucleus, or central atom, of wheatgrass juice is magnesium, and the nucleus of hemoglobin, our blood, is iron. Dr. Jeffrey Dach is board certified in diagnostic and interventional radiology and board certified with the American Academy of Anti-Aging Medicine. (Dach "Wheatgrass" 2013)

Wheatgrass juice carries oxygen and alkalinity to our cells. This helps our cells repair, rebuild and become functional once again. Wheatgrass juice is loaded with antioxidants. Free radicals (unidentified flying objects) in our body, which our body doesn't know how to assimilate, are always present. With so much air and water pollution, electro-magnetic and radiation exposure, not to mention the SAD diet we consume, it's almost impossible to avoid free radicals unless you live in a bubble. Since wheatgrass juice is loaded with antioxidants, it destroys free radicals, which contribute, in a huge way, to aging.

If you want the real fountain of youth, it's wheatgrass juice. Wheatgrass planting, growing and harvesting instructions are included in the Appendix.

Jim Miller recovered from non-Hodgkin's leukemic lymphoma, thought by most of the medical profession as incurable, by using a raw-food diet and vegetable juicing, particularly wheatgrass juice and sunflower sprouts. He did this even after receiving six cycles of chemotherapy. Sunflower sprouts are loaded with nutrients and antioxidants just like wheatgrass juice, and they are thirty-five times more nutritious than broccoli. His story is included in the chapter of testimonials.

Jim's message is phenomenal, and he believes that juicing wheatgrass and eating sunflower sprouts were two of the main reasons he recovered completely. Jim also produced a YouTube video showing how to grow wheatgrass. (Miller "How to Grow Wheatgrass – Jim Miller" 2012)

Wheatgrass also contains chlorophyll, which increases hemoglobin production, and selenium and laetrile, both of which help to restore our immune system. More oxygen gets to the cancer cells, and since cancer cannot live in an oxygenated environment, it helps to annihilate cancer cells.

When you juice any fruit or vegetable it needs to be consumed right away or at least within ten to twenty minutes of juicing so you get the maximum benefit from the enzymes. You can also refrigerate juices in airtight, dark, glass or thermos-like containers and consume them throughout the day, but fresh is still best. As fresh juice is exposed to the heat, air, and light, it begins to oxidize, meaning it loses its nutritional value very quickly. As you drink fresh juice on an empty stomach, it's absorbed into your bloodstream immediately, causing the enzymes and nutrients to get right to work at repairing your cells and returning them to a healthy and whole state. Canned and bottled juices have been heated to kill any bacteria or viruses present in the juice's raw state and to provide shelf life. When this happens, the enzymes are destroyed. Remember, anything cooked is dead food. Drinking fresh juices is like getting an intravenous infusion of immunity. It's that powerful.

Clean, Pure Water and Air

I mentioned our water and air problems earlier, so I won't get into those details again. It's enough to say please get a water-purification system for your home and some kind of heavy-duty air cleaner to attach to your heating and air conditioning system.

Water/Coffee Enemas

I've heard all kinds of people talk about how awful and disgusting enemas are. The mere thought of it makes people cringe. You want me to what? You want me to lie on the floor and insert a little white plastic tip into my anus, followed by a couple of quarts of water? Then you want me to release the water and repeat the process, but this time with one quart of coffee or some other healing liquid? And then I lay there for between ten and twenty minutes? *Huh?*

Well, is being sick and diseased any less disgusting? How disgusting do your insides look from all the years of toxic waste build-up? If you smoke, I'm sure your lungs could use an overhaul. Is undergoing chemotherapy, radiation, and additional surgery any less disgusting than being in the comfort of your own home administering to your own care with healing techniques that work without caustic side effects? Have you been diagnosed with terminal cancer, diabetes, heart disease, or any other disease that is going to make you run to the undertaker to start making plans for your *final* arrangements?

I'll bet enemas are beginning to sound incredibly harmless right now, aren't they? I'd rather be lying flat on my bathroom floor giving myself an enema than lying flat in a hospital bed at some clinic with a needle in my vein giving me a dose of useless, ineffective, poisonous, chemotherapy that will just make my hair fall out, cause me to be tired all the time, make me nauseous, and cause vomiting—or, worse yet, lying dead with formaldehyde in my veins, inside a double-vaulted rectangular box, six feet under the ground with a headstone bearing my name.

Enemas are a healing mechanism for your body with no caustic side effects. Are you listening? Is anyone hearing this? A clean colon is one of the basic elements necessary to maintain optimum health. Your colon harbors hundreds of types of both friendly and unfriendly bacteria, and when those bacteria get out of balance, the colon does not work properly.

When you consume a diet high in animal fats, sugar, and processed foods, you're most likely not getting the fiber you need to brush the colon clean on a daily basis. When that happens, food begins to get stuck in the colon pockets and walls and can lead to diverticulosis and Crohn's Disease, among other diseases.

I've said it before, and I'll say it again. I know people who were diagnosed with stage-four cancer with just a couple of months to live who completely recovered using alternatives. Jim Miller is just one of them. One of these alternatives is the use of enemas for detoxing the body from the toxic overload that got you into this diseased state to begin with.

I know this may sound crazy, but I must say that giving myself enemas twice a day during that one week a month when I did a juice fast was some of the most spiritual and precious time of my day. Here's how I made it work for me.

First, I lit an essential oil candle to bring peace and light into the bathroom. The candle aroma was calming and healing for me. Then I took out my coconut oil, or you can get a vegetable based non-petroleum jelly to put on the white plastic tip going inside you. Then I got my reading glasses, the most recent book I was reading, and my watch. I put a comfortable mat (like a yoga mat) on the bathroom floor, covered by a large bath or beach towel, and brought in my bed pillow and a blanket. Sometimes I played soft gentle healing music in the background.

Since the water enema is the fastest one, I just put the water in and then went to release it. When it was coffee time, I lay down, made myself comfortable and put the coffee in. Then I covered myself up with my warm wool blanket, put my head on my fluffy soft pillow, got cozy, picked up my book, looked at my watch, and started to read whatever health or spiritual book I was reading at the time. Before I started to read I always visualized this process healing me, cleaning my liver and gall bladder, causing these organs to release more toxins. I visualized myself as whole again, well again, cancer free, and living life to the fullest.

Sometimes, I just meditated on those same aspects during the whole twenty minutes. With my eyes closed I created this vision of all my bodily organs operating at peak efficiency, toxin free, with the juicing, supplements, and organic raw food diet I was consuming creating strength and vitality where there was none before. This was the best twenty minutes of my day then. Can you see how this could be a special time for you, too?

Always do the water enema first, as this is when you wash out the toxins that accumulated in your colon overnight, and you don't want to reabsorb them. You're on a cleaning spree here. After the coffee goes in, you lie on your left or right side. At HealthQuarters they suggested the left side. Other healing centers suggest the right side. I think either side is fine, as both ascending and descending colon sections have large arteries attached which extend from those areas to the liver. The coffee is absorbed through the colon wall and taken up to the liver by the artery. The caffeine stimulates the liver and gallbladder to contract, causing them to release yet more toxins. This is part of the detox process that is ever-so-necessary in any healing process. Check with your own alternative health-care practitioner for their suggestions, and don't go "cold turkey" without consulting with someone who can guide you through this process. Detoxing is not for the faint of heart.

After your ten or twenty minutes are up, go and release the coffee. I knew this would take a few minutes, so I brought my book in with me to prevent boredom from the amount of time it took to empty out. To move this process along a little more quickly, you can take your hand, palm side down, and gently move it from the lower part of your ascending colon (along the right side of your body) to the top of it (about the location of your belly button or waist). Then move your hand across from the top of the ascending colon to the left of your body across the entire transverse colon. When you get to the other side, move your hand down the left side of your body from the top of the descending colon down to the bottom of it. In essence this creates an upside down U- shaped movement. This helps to move the liquid up and out a little more quickly. Be gentle with yourself.

When you feel empty, praise yourself for a job well done and know for certain that you are being healed. Have no question in your mind about it. Banish all doubt! The best part is that *you* are doing it for yourself without any negative side effects or consequences. You just feel so good all over. Ooooohhh. Can't wait until the next one! And you won't feel like having that real cup of coffee either!

Make sure you thoroughly disinfect all your *tools* with antibacterial soap. Every once in a while you can use a very mild bleach and water solution to clean the plastic parts. We'll get into some detox surprises from these enemas in the next chapter.

Liver-Gallbladder Flush

Your liver, what's it used for? It's the largest internal organ in your body and its functions are many. One is to filter your blood. So imagine your liver acting like a car or home air conditioner. What happens when these filters get obstructed with grease, dirt, and dust particles? The car or home air conditioners no longer work at peak efficiency, and the air in your car and home starts to get stuffy and doesn't smell quite as nice as it used to. The clogged up filters also put extra stress and strain on the air conditioners trying to produce clean, pure air for you to breathe.

Almost the same thing happens with your liver. When it gets a traffic jam of excessive grease (fat), dirt, and dust (sugars, salts, and other toxins), it doesn't work so well. There's just one problem with your liver, you can't just to go to a big box store, the local hardware store, or the auto supply store, purchase a new liver, and change it out.

When we don't nourish our body with healthy food, moderate exercise, restful sleep, and pure, clean water, our liver and other organs start to malfunction. When that happens we can be in for many serious immune system problems and failures. My problems and failures were surely rearing their ugly heads.

Your gallbladder, what's it used for? It stores bile made by your liver to aid in the digestion of fats. When you eat so much fat, and so much of the wrong kind of fats, your liver and gallbladder can't make enough bile to keep the digestion process going. The excess fat finds its way into your bloodstream and ends up collecting in your liver and arteries and can appear as large clusters of cholesterol deposits.

When your liver can't take it any more, the undigested fats also accumulate in your gallbladder, and then we have such things as fatty-liver disease and gallstones, sometimes leading your doctor to recommend that your gallbladder be removed. How sad when most of the time you just need a few rounds of flushes, a change in your diet, more exercise, and, presto! No surgery. You just saved a very important organ in your body.

I emotionally beat up on myself pretty badly while I was in Colorado Springs. I started to question myself, how my mother prepared food for us, and how my grandmother prepared food for her family. All this time I realized the mistakes I previously made. Well, I would no longer be making them. My food preparation methods were going to change. I had a wake-up call. I heard it loud and clear, and I was going make some real, positive changes in all areas of my health. This whole experience could have been avoided if I made better choices earlier on, but I just didn't know any better; no one taught me any other way.

Even home economics, as it was called when I was in high school, didn't share this kind of information. It was the old FDA food pyramid back then. The schools were just teaching what the government was telling them to teach.

So on the evening of the fourth day at HealthQuarters we did a liver-gallbladder flush. Again my eyebrows went up and my eyes got wide with wonder, but I was committed to this program so I was going to follow it to the letter.

A liver-gallbladder flush does the same thing as an enema in terms of releasing toxins, but this time I was going to get rid of gallstones and large cholesterol deposits that have been clogging up my liver and gallbladder, preventing those filters from operating at peak efficiency.

The preparation for a liver-gallbladder flush takes a bit longer, but is also very cleansing and healing. For the best results do this when you're doing a juice fast and over a long weekend when you have time to rest and not be distracted.

First you take a couple of magnesium malate capsules three times a day and/or drink two cups of freshly made apple juice, diluted 50 percent with pure water, twice a day. The malic acid in the apple juice and the magnesium malate help to soften any gallstones and cholesterol deposits. Do this for four days.

In the meantime, purchase a bottle of magnesium citrate at the pharmacy. It comes in lemon and cherry flavors. Go to your local health-food store and pick up a bottle of organic lemon juice and a bottle of organic, extra-virgin, first-cold-pressed olive oil. For this procedure you don't need fresh lemon juice, but you could make it if you wanted to. Your grocery store may carry all these items, now that each one usually has a pharmacy department. Grocery stores are beginning to carry more organic products now, also.

On the evening of the fourth day, around 7:00 p.m., mix two ounces of olive oil and four ounces of lemon juice. You can use an electric hand blender for the mixing so the oil and the lemon juice are more consistently mixed. Drink it down quickly. I know you're saying *yuck* again, right? It really was OK, at least for me. I was on a mission; it had to be OK.

Immediately after you drink this mixture, lie down on your right side and pull your right knee up to your chest as far as it will comfortably go for about twenty to thirty minutes. This opens the pathway to your gallbladder and allows the lemon and olive oil to flow easily into your gallbladder so it can get in there and do the work. The work is to cause the liver and gallbladder to contract and spit out the gallstones, cholesterol deposits, and toxins into your digestive tract.

You may feel a bit of nausea, but that's all. You shouldn't feel any discomfort from the gallstones leaving the liver or gallbladder; it's literally quite painless.

Rest during this time, lie down, read a good book, watch a good movie, but rest. Around 9:00 p.m. begin to drink that ten-ounce bottle of magnesium citrate and drink as much as you can. You can also make an Epsom Salt version of this drink in the event the magnesium citrate doesn't go down too well. Of course, you can follow this drink with some pure water. The magnesium citrate or the Epsom Salt solution helps to move the toxins quickly through your intestines so they don't get reabsorbed. This was the most unpleasant part of the process for me. But down it went, every last drop, followed by a lot of water.

Remember to do your morning enema, even if you already had your bowel movement at some point during the night. This part is very important, because you will be washing out toxins accumulated during the night, and you want to keep moving these toxins out of your body. You don't want to reabsorb them. How do you know the toxins are moving out of your body? You begin to feel better, and better, and better!

The gallstones that were in my liver and gallbladder were just some of the problems with my body not functioning properly and at peak efficiency. Again, this *seeing is believing* part of my recovery was like another slap in the face. We'll talk more about the results in the chapter on Detox Surprises.

Supplements

We've been told that as we age we begin to lose our mental and physical faculties. Take a look at our diets: toaster pastries for breakfast, fast food for lunch, microwavable processed food for dinner. Where is the nutrition? Practically *zero* in all of these meals. Our bodies are living organisms, and we need to eat live food in order to sustain this physical aspect of who we are. A recent TV commercial I saw when I was rebounding showed a woman having what looked like a bowl of granola for breakfast. You know, one serving equals just about a tablespoon. A man dressed like the sun was present to share a different breakfast strategy with her, a microwavable sausage, egg, and cheese sandwich. Yum, she says as she bites into it with a huge smile on her face. See how they can hook you? Anyway, the sun had done its job, and she finishes the sandwich and goes to work. The sun places the bowl of granola on the windowsill, and the birds are now perched on the edge of the bowl picking at the cereal.

The whole idea was that both breakfast items contained less than 300 calories. In my opinion, 300 calories or not, there was next to zero nutrition, both meals loaded with chemicals. Yes, some granolas are not the healthy food you think they are. You can make a quick green smoothie loaded with all kinds of nutrition for way under 300 calories and with zero chemicals. What's wrong with this picture? You don't see any TV ads for green smoothies. People just don't know they have incredibly healthy, low cost, easy to prepare, options available to them, so they become pawns of the processed world, whether it's granola, microwavable sandwiches, or frozen pizzas.

Any food cooked over 118 degrees is considered mostly void of any nutritional value. So if you have lived a lifetime of eating processed food and food void of any nutritional value, then of course your body is going to deteriorate. But it doesn't have to, and you can recover. I am living proof of this, and so are many other people who have similar stories to share.

We've all been victims, and I really dislike using that term anymore, but it fits in this case. We've fallen prey to the pharmaceutical and processed food manufacturers' worlds through marketing and advertising. At one time or another we've all been sold a bill of goods, exchanging our health for the convenience and speed of getting meals on the table so that we've forgotten what real food tastes like.

I suggest to you, without a morsel of doubt, that real, organic, raw or even some organic, cooked food tastes *great*. The reason you don't like real food is that your taste buds have been neutered by all the chemicals, poisons, food additives, and preservatives in processed food. These chemicals have seriously altered your taste buds, not to mention what the interior of your body must look and feel like.

The food manufacturing industry puts all these additives into their processed food in an attempt to get and keep you addicted to all processed food they manufacture. Then you age, get diseases of all kinds, and wonder why. Why? Because you're filled with toxic chemicals. Your body is crying out for the life-sustaining organic, raw fruits and vegetables Mother Nature created that will keep you vibrantly healthy for a very long foreseeable future. I've already talked about MSG and the related names it can be processed into, but another one is aspartame, an artificial sweetener.

These additives are used in large measure to make food taste *better* or to reduce calorie count in processed food. Of course processed food requires additives in order to make it taste better because it's been so over processed that it's tasteless and lifeless. Because these additives are void of any nutrition you want to eat more and more of this lifeless food so you can feel full. So your body remains starved even though your stomach is now stretched to excess. Processed food manufacturers get you hooked through marketing and advertising. Then you become addicted, buy more, eat more, and feel full but are terribly unsatisfied nutritionally. Then you get fat, diseased, and sometimes die.

We may be living longer, but in what state of health? Modern medicine has allowed us to have a higher longevity rate, but at what expense? Is it a good thing to be alive while unable to really live, spending the last years of life in a vegetative state, in a chair or bed, unable to move? The drugs you take may be slowly and painfully killing you. Are you traveling? Are you experiencing the love of your families? Are you dancing, loving, and living your dreams and your passions? Are you doing what you want to do in your later years? Do you want to live the last years of your life from a lonely room in an assisted-living center, sitting in a wheelchair, blankly staring out a window, not knowing your family or friends? This does not have to happen. You can live a different life. I want to live, love, dance and let death wait for me.

Supplements helped me restore and rebuild my immune system while I was changing my diet and lifestyle. The problem is that so many of us take what we think we need by way of advertising that we could be taking unnecessarily an excess of some supplements and not actually taking enough of some others. It's really best to work with an alternative-health-care specialist who can perform muscle response testing (MRT) on your body to assess its nutritional and supplemental needs. That person can also guide you to purchase organic-quality, whole-food, vitamin and mineral supplements.

I remember once going to a health expo, where there was a host of supplement companies marketing and selling their products. When I opened the container of some of these vitamin bottles, the stench was overwhelming. It reeked of chemicals. Organic, whole-food vitamin supplements will not smell like this. They're made from real, whole food, not chemical substitutes.

The truth is that sometimes you can be fooled by the product manufacturers' quantities measured in milligrams or grams. Say one brand, we'll call it the intruder, is offering a vitamin C supplement in doses of ten-thousand milligrams. The organic, whole-food vitamin C supplement dose is only two thousand milligrams. You may think that if two thousand milligrams is good, ten-thousand milligrams is better, right? The whole-food vitamin C costs more and contains eight-thousand fewer milligrams than the intruder vitamin C. So you think you'll get more bang for your buck buying the intruder, right?

Once again, your body does not necessarily recognize or absorb all ten-thousand milligrams of the intruder vitamin C because it can't. It may not be from a calcium source your body can regognize. Your body absorbs and uses all two-thousand milligrams of the organic, whole-food vitamin C because it really is *all natural*, and your body knows what to do with real whole food.

Your alternative-health-care provider can steer you in the right direction.

Exercise

You cannot get from sickness to health without some form of exercise. I'm fairly certain that part of the reason why you got sick, if you are sick, is because the TV has had you addicted to it. No, you don't have to pump, push, pull, or press anything hard to exercise, unless that's your choice. You do need to move your body every day to move the toxins from your lymph system. Your lymph system has no pump associated with it, like the blood in your veins, which is moved by your heart pump. We have no way to move lymph fluid unless we move it by way of exercise.

Your lymph system is a series of nodes located in various parts of your body which collect toxic waste. When you exercise, these nodes release the toxins, and the toxins are flushed from your body. If you don't exercise, your lymph nodes accumulate toxins until an overload occurs, which can result in various kinds of disease, cancer being just one of them.

Yes, everyone says that walking is good exercise, and it certainly is, but can't you find something that's as good or better that you positively love to do? For me it's dancing. I wanted to dance my whole life, and I seldom did. I now take private and group lessons three times a week, and then I'm dancing at various venues three or four times a week, too. The pure truth of it is, dancing is in my blood, and I would rather dance than eat. I love to waltz, foxtrot, tango, rumba, cha cha, salsa and swing!

While I do my domestic goddess duties in or around the house or when I'm writing, I always have some kind of music on in the background. I'm passionate about many different types of music. It moves me, speaks to my soul, inspires me, and fills me up; I even dance in my chair sometimes when I'm working on the computer.

Dancing is also a great way to feel connected with another human being, holding hands, being wrapped in another's arms, feeling the other's energy as you move around the dance floor. Try it, you'll like it! Dancing is much better than walking and certainly much better than watching depressing TV programs, many filled with some kind of violence.

The point is to find some physical activity you *love* to do and have a passion for, and you'll never have to exercise, ever again. You'll never have to see the inside of a gym anywhere, ever, unless you like working out at a gym. Dancing or other sporting activities also provide an opportunity for social interaction, getting connected with people of like minds, enjoying stimulating conversation, and living! I can't tell you how many wonderful people I've connected with since I started dancing.

There is actually some research to indicate ballroom dancing in particular is actually a great way of not only physically exercising, but also making you smarter by increasing the cognitive pathways in the brain which, as you age, disappear. By now you know that I believe aging is primarily a result of bad diets and lifestyles, and not just because we're getting older. Being a huge fan of dancing, I just had to include some excerpts from this article by Richard Powers. The research was really clear on the multiple benefits of ballroom dancing.

From "Use It or Lose It: Dancing Makes You Smarter":

> For centuries, dance manuals and other writings have lauded the health benefits of dancing, usually as physical exercise. More recently we've seen research on further health benefits of dancing, such as stress reduction and increased serotonin level, with its sense of well-being.

> Then most recently we've heard of another benefit: Frequent dancing apparently makes us smarter. A major study added to the growing evidence that stimulating one's mind can ward off Alzheimer's disease and other dementia, much as physical exercise can keep the body fit. Dancing also increases cognitive acuity at all ages. (Stanford "Use It or Lose It: Dancing Makes You Smarter" 2010)

The article goes into some depth about the details of the research, but it sums up like this. Ballroom dancing scores the highest in cognitive results because it requires the brain to quickly make split-second determinations regarding movement. Both the lead and follow roles benefit because each party makes rapid fire decisions in order to dance cohesively to the beat and rhythm of the music. More is better in this case. Do it at least three to four times a week, but as much as you can if that is not possible.

You can discover more about Richard Powers at his website. (Powers 2010)

Rebounding

A mini-trampoline can give you the benefit of about an hour's worth of exercise in just about ten to twenty minutes. A mini-trampoline, also called a rebounder, is about three feet wide and resembles a larger trampoline that you've seen children use in their backyard playgrounds, only this one is small enough to use inside your home—in your living room, garage, bedroom, or anywhere space permits both vertically and horizontally. All you do is get on it and jump gently or not so gently, depending on how comfortable you get with it. This device also has a removable handlebar that you can take off once you've established your balance, or leave on if that's your preference.

The benefits of rebounding are immense. Here are just some of them:
- increases capacity for respiration
- increases oxygen to every cell of your body
- aids in lymphatic circulation and detoxification
- enhances digestion and elimination processes
- promotes body growth and repair
- exercises your muscles with very little effort
- promotes blood flow to the smallest of capillaries for repair and regeneration of surrounding tissue
- reduces stress

I rebound three to four times a week, in addition to all the dancing I do. As I mentioned before, I do this while watching an episode of HGTV, so the time goes by quickly. Rebounders are an inexpensive way to reboot your body's systems into functioning again if you've been sedentary for a very long time. Purchase a good quality rebounder and you'll have it for life. You have to keep your body moving. Movement means life is present. Without movement, life doesn't exist.

Soaks and Saunas

A sauna causes you to sweat. Sweat causes you to detoxify through the pores of your skin. I was very fortunate in that I had a whirlpool tub and a sauna in my previous home. I used them regularly, even before I had a reason to.

With the sauna temperature warmed up to around 150 degrees, I would sweat like crazy. I would stay in there for about fifteen minutes, sometimes longer if I could stand it. I enjoy dry heat and so it felt really good.

When I was finished, I would take a whirlpool bath. The difference between a whirlpool bath and a spa or hot tub is one word, chemicals. A spa or hot tub requires you to keep the water in the hot tub indefinitely, and you do this is by chemically treating the water so bacteria won't grow. Well, chemicals usually mean some kind of chlorine, and chlorine is very toxic. Think about this for a second. When you get into a hot tub, the temperature is around 100 degrees. This will open the pores all over your body, and the chlorine and other chemicals used to treat the water are going to be absorbed into your body through your skin. You're trying to get rid of toxic chemicals, not add more.

When you take a whirlpool bath you change the water every time. You also have the ability to add some de-chlorinating bath salts, Epsom salts, and essential oils for relaxation and fragrance. The gentle heat of the water and the whirlpool action help to stimulate lymph flow and relax your muscles and other organs so you can unwind and get a better night's sleep. This *treatment* is like going to a spa, and it does wonders to support the healing process. I would take saunas and soaks about three times a week.

Dry Skin Brushing

The skin is an organ, the largest eliminative organ of the body, also sometimes called the third kidney. The skin can eliminate more than a pound of waste products in the form of sweat throughout the day. Are you drinking enough water? The skin is also an absorptive organ. The skin absorbs oxygen, vitamins, minerals, and even protein as well as it can absorb toxic substances, which then find their way into other organs.

Yes, even the laundry detergent and fabric softener we think has been rinsed out of our clothes and particles from artificial fabrics are absorbed into our body through our skin. Hand and body lotions clog our pores and prevent our skin from detoxing naturally through sweat. Try washing your hands with pure castile soap, so soft and gentle. It smells great, too. You'll never use other brands again.

Dry skin brushing is based upon the ancient Chinese concepts of acupuncture and acupressure. According to the Chinese, there are three million nerve points spread over the surface of the skin, seven hundred of which are nodal. Stimulation of these nodal points causes current flow through channels called meridians and either stimulate or suppress the activity of specific organs to which they are connected. For example, a point between the thumb and forefinger of the right hand connects to the liver.

By applying friction to the acupuncture points, dry skin brushing is designed to take advantage of these countless connections. The entire nervous system is stimulated and invigorated, and every organ, gland, muscle and ligament benefits.

Dry skin brushing, if done in the correct fashion, also helps to physically remove toxic lymph fluid through the lymph vessels toward the central venous circulation system so that toxins in the lymph fluid and in the tissues can be cleared from the body by other toxin-clearing organs, including the kidneys, liver, intestines, and lungs.

Use only a natural bristle brush, which you can buy online, from a health-food store, now even some drug stores, or grocery store pharmacies. The bristles range from softer to firmer, depending on your particular skin sensitivity. Dry skin brushing is very invigorating and makes your skin feel softer than any lotion you can buy. It accomplishes this by getting rid of dead skin cells at the surface level, unclogging your pores, and allowing your skin to breathe again.

Here's a YouTube video that demonstrates just how to perform this exercise. (Owens "The correct way to skin brush!" 2011)

Sleep

Sleep rebuilds, repairs, and restores. Sleep is a time when your body and mind relax from the day's activities, and no detoxification program would be complete without the need for restful, uninterrupted sleep.

Your body goes through three stages during the day in approximately eight-hour intervals: elimination, appropriation, and assimilation.

Elimination takes place usually between the hours of 4:00 a.m. and 12:00 noon. This is the time when your body eliminates waste products and toxins through your bowels.

Appropriation is your meal intake during the day. As your body takes in nutrition and begins the digestion process, it is also preparing for the next stage of assimilation. The appropriation cycle generally occurs between 12:00 noon and 8:00 p.m.

Assimilation takes place when your body takes the nutrition you took in during the appropriation stage and begins to repair, rebuild, and restore your body's systems during the night. This stage occurs from around 8:00 p.m. to 4:00 a.m.

In preparation for sleep you may want to avoid eating anything after 7:00 or 8:00 p.m. or earlier. Since 70 to 80 percent of your body's energy is devoted to digestion, eating a meal late at night will surely keep you awake because your body won't be resting, it will be digesting. Digestion is a big job for your body during the day, and late at night it's worse yet. Your body is tired and wants to sleep, not begin what could be a very painstaking job.

Alcohol can make you drowsy for sure, but it never is a way to obtain good sleep. On the rare occasion when I have a cocktail at night, even if it's in the early evening, I just don't sleep as well as on those nights when I have no alcohol at all. Certainly avoid drinking a lot of water just before bed. We all know this can cause a need to use the bathroom in the middle of the night, and this can dramatically interrupt your ability to get back to sleep and into the peaceful place you woke from.

Avoid exercising late, too. Your body will be over stimulated, and it could take hours for you to calm down and get to a place where restful sleep can occur.

You may also want to try some meditation just before going to bed, taking some deep cleansing breaths and releasing any tension left from your day. Say your prayers; send blessings to those you love and even more to the ones who challenge you. These are the people who cause you to grow. Be grateful, thankful, and appreciative of the people, places, and events that got you through your day. A simple state of appreciation relaxes me because it's a feel-good experience. Say ahh!

Now go have some pleasant dreams.

Read the Labels

If you can't pronounce the ingredients on the product label, chances are it's something you don't want in or on you. Read the advisories or warnings about the product. If it has a warning label of any kind, chances are it is loaded with toxic chemicals, especially if it has a skull and crossbones on it, warns of calling the poison control center, rushing to the emergency room, or inducing vomiting if accidentally swallowed.

Anything with the letters prop or propyl usually means its source is oil or some type of petroleum product. Do we really want these things in our bodies?

There is an interesting article published in the October 2006 issue of *National Geographic* magazine (which is now online) titled "Chemicals Within Us" by David Ewing Duncan. Duncan discusses interesting ideas about various toxins, where we get them, and how we can or can't get rid of them. The article leads us to believe that we may not be able to get rid of some of them. Poppycock! There is always a way. (National "Chemicals Within Us" 2013)

CHAPTER **8**

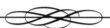

Detox Surprises

I HOPE YOU DON'T BECOME GROSSED out by the information and pictures I'll share with you in this chapter. It may come as a huge surprise to you that we all get or have parasites, may have thick gooey stuff stuck on our intestinal walls, and may be harboring gallstones and cholesterol deposits of mass proportions, contributing to our being sick and diseased. You may have one or all of these things right now, so it's important for you to know how these disease promoters enter your body and how to eliminate them, as well as to learn some prevention steps necessary to minimize their return.

Impacted Fecal Matter

I wasn't expecting to see anything unusual on this day, just the normal enema routine. However, on the fifth day at HealthQuarters, I began my day with the usual water enema first thing in the morning—I filled up the hot water bottle, lay down on the floor to begin, and in went the water, all eight cups. Then, as I was required, I went to the toilet to let out the water. *Surprise!* I just love talking about this part of my program because what came out was such a *huge* surprise to me. In this case, seeing was believing. I felt this big ker-plunk into the toilet, along with a big backsplash. I stopped the discharge of the water from my colon and got up to look around and see what was there, and I couldn't believe my eyes.

I called to my sister Patti, "You've got to take a look at this!"

Yes, we are that close that we could do this and feel comfortable with each other about it, especially knowing the reason we were doing this program in the first place. She couldn't believe it either. We found a way to fish it out of the toilet and put it in a plastic cup without touching it and started poking at it.

It was about a foot long (no, we're not talking about a hot dog here), a half inch wide, dense, dark brown almost black, impacted fecal matter, which looked very much like a big strand of pearls. I didn't know what it was then, but I sure found out quickly enough. It was almost "show and tell" at class that day. I kept poking at it in total disbelief. It was rubbery to the touch. No, I didn't touch it with my hands, but with my poking tool. I think it was a plastic knife, spoon or something like that. I kept poking and poking and moving it around in the cup, and still I wondered where this stuff came from in my body. My sister did the same thing, poking and prodding it, wondering what it was and from where in my body this originated. This *crap* came out of my body? At the same time I was observing this disgusting, yet fascinating, substance, I knew, I just knew, that this entire process was going to get and keep me well.

What incredible things I learned about impacted fecal matter: how it starts, how it can be eliminated, and why it's detrimental to your health. Here's my interpretation of what I believe to be the evolution of my own impacted fecal matter.

Evolution of Impacted Fecal Matter (At Least Mine)

This stuff doesn't just accumulate overnight; it takes years. My problem involved the following: too much meat, dairy, cheese, milk, ice cream, butter, sugary treats (I used to love making homemade apple pie with a real Crisco crust), eating way too much at each meal, and not eating nearly enough fiber. With all that fat, there's no room for fiber, right? When you overeat at every meal, your stomach has a hard time digesting all that food, and it slowly moves through your small intestine and eventually into your large intestine, your colon. Did I say slowly? Imagine eating every meal as if it were your last. What could possibly be the consequences of eating excessively at every meal? Cancer, that's what, and so many other diseases, too. So I believe the beginning of my health problem dates back to my childhood Doritos and Oreo days. Bad habits are hard to break, and although I was able to let go of Oreos, I still ate plenty of Doritos, in my previous life.

By the way, you can find all kinds of information on the Internet about impacted fecal matter, and don't be surprised if there are some reports that say this just isn't true. There are contradictions, even in alternative medicine. But as I said, seeing is believing, and this experience made a believer out of me. While I don't have pictures of the original *ker-plunk* from my experience at HealthQuarters in Colorado, here are some pictures of a section that came out of me during a recent cleanse.

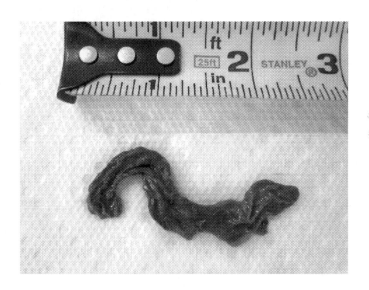

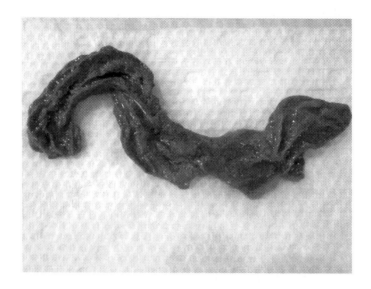

Yes, of course I poked and prodded it. It had a thick, rubbery texture, indicating it probably had been in there quite some time, and I perform a detox or a cleanse of some kind about every six months or so. You can see in the close-up picture above, the folds, nooks, and crannies. In my opinion this was caused by undigested dairy. It just stuck to the walls of my intestines and took on the shape and nature of that intestinal section.

Imagine what your own impacted fecal matter may look like if you've never done a colon cleanse, with all that undigested food roaming around in your intestines. Even though my diet is relatively clean, you can see what happens when you know a certain food doesn't work for you and you decide to eat it any way. I know I shouldn't eat cheese and other dairy products, but I'm human and occasionally do indulge. I got back into the habit of drinking one cup of coffee in the morning with half and half and infrequently eating some parmesan cheese on organic brown rice or quinoa pastas. I believe this impacted fecal matter was a direct result of undigested dairy.

The moral of my story is, don't do dairy—at all! It just sticks to your insides and can wreak havoc with your health. Just imagine if I didn't perform a periodic cleanse how this could build up in my colon once again.

For many of us, eating meat puts our digestive system under great stress. Animal protein of any kind usually digests slowly, and our bodies are not designed to consume or digest meat. Our teeth and enzymes cannot break down the animal proteins into small enough particles to be safely digested and utilized properly. Meat can also ferment in our digestive system because of the slow processing speed. As part of our Standard American Diet, meat is usually eaten with some kind of white carbohydrate like potatoes, rice, pasta, or bread. If you're going to eat meat, I suggest you consume it with green vegetables and salad. Take a look at this video. The presenter humorously discusses the benefits of a plant-based diet. (Real Food Channel "The Best Diet" 2012)

Eat brown carbohydrates like whole wheat pasta, brown rice, or potatoes with veggies. Save the fruit for one half hour before a meal or an hour or more after a meal. Fruit should only be eaten alone on an empty stomach. The natural sugar in fruit and the normal quick digestion process causes it to slow down when other food is also present and processing, so the sugar causes fermentation. Adding fruit to a main meal can be disastrous, creating intestinal distress, flatulence, and the slow digestion that can put extra stress on the lining of the intestines.

There's a food-combining guide that shows us what types of food to combine with others for the best digestion and utilization of nutrients. Check out the Internet for some options on where to get one and read all about how this simple yet powerful food-combining plan can save your digestive system from becoming overwhelmed, shut down, and possibly cause an illness.

Picture This

Our intestines have two walls, an interior wall and an exterior wall. If you put too much air into a balloon, what happens? It breaks. Now imagine two balloons, one smaller one inside a larger one. The inside balloon is filled with a toxic substance (undigested fermenting food) and is stretched so much that it breaks. Now we have a break in the interior wall of the intestine. When that happens, undigested fermenting food particles leak through and settle in between the walls of the two balloons, our intestinal walls. This creates a hiding place for undigested food particles. How do you know you have a tear in the wall of the inside balloon, the intestinal lining? Maybe you start feeling a bit tired or lethargic, but nothing serious enough to put you down or cause you to see your doctor. So it's back to meal time, business as usual, overeating the same SAD food in the wrong combinations. Guess what happens next? More food gets very slowly processed through the intestinal wall and lodges between the inside and outside walls of the intestinal lining.

This process never stops because you just don't know what's happening to you. You start to get a big belly, your bathroom scale shows signs of weight increase, and you need to go shopping for the next bigger size of whatever you're wearing. That by itself should be a warning signal, but, again, you're just putting on some extra pounds. You could justify this by saying, "I'm getting older." Obesity in this country is rampant among both adults and young children. Old people get fat and sick just by virtue of the fact that they're older, right? I don't think so. What's happening to the younger folks who are in their teens, twenties, thirties, and forties? What's their excuse?

Over time, the undigested food particles accumulate as they are lodged in between the intestinal walls. The food begins to rot, and your intestines get more stretched out with every meal and store larger and larger quantities of undigested food. It has nowhere to go, so what happens? It becomes hard and takes on the shape and form of the intestinal location. As more and more stress is put on the outside balloon, the outer lining of the intestine can break. If it does, now your intestinal walls have been completely damaged and compromised to the point where you begin to auto-intoxicate with all kinds of undigested food particles, proteins, and poop that are trapped between the inside lining and the outside lining. Now this toxic material is actually being re-absorbed into your body, and you have what is referred to as leaky-gut syndrome. The inside and outside walls are torn. Clearly you can see how this condition can reduce the ability of any nutrients in your food to reach your bloodstream. Now you begin to feel symptoms that really do make you sick—stomach pain, fatigue, and bloating, among others. Now you really are sick, have a seriously impacted colon, and need to visit the doctor to find out why.

But wait, where do the parasites come in? The parasites have now passed by the hydrochloric acid in your stomach on their way through your intestines and find a warm fuzzy place to nest. Many of us don't produce enough hydrochloric acid which can be the first line of defense against parasites and can help break down food once it enters our stomach. Parasites find their way through the break in the intestinal lining and feed on the impacted fecal matter. In fact, they like it so much they begin to attach themselves to the intestinal lining, thereby creating a really nice hold inside your belly.

During this process you can accumulate all kinds of both microscopic parasites and larger ones like tapeworms. Seventy percent or more (depending on the source) of your immune system is in your gut. So if you have a wall of rotting meat and other food particles trapped between your food and your bloodstream, what's getting through to sustain you? Not much, if anything. No wonder so many people with big bellies are very sick, not just obese.

Some of you have wounds that won't heal and a whole host of other daily problems like colds, flu, allergies, asthma, and bronchial infections, just to name a few. You just aren't getting the nutrient density you need from your food to keep you alive, especially if you aren't eating the right kinds of foods in the first place.

People say to me all the time, "I just had a colonoscopy, so I'm sure I don't have any of that stuff in me."

I had a colonoscopy, too, before I was diagnosed with cancer. I learned that just because you've been cleared out of the obvious stuff inside your colon doesn't mean the accumulation lodged in between the walls of your intestines has been cleaned out. Remember, like the cockroach, the parasites taking up residence are pretty strong, and their will to survive is even stronger, and you're giving them plenty of life-sustaining sugar, salt, and fat, if you're still eating a Standard American Diet. They hang on because they're fat and happy there. They live long and colonize until something comes along to really knock them off their feet.

Para-Cleanse by Nature's Sunshine to the rescue! The Para-Cleanse ingredients were combined with parasites in mind and can reach these little buggers like a can of Raid for your body. By the way, I never once felt sick, nauseous, distressed or uneasy taking Para-Cleanse, with all of its strange ingredients. In fact, the more evidence I got from this cleanse, the better I felt inside and looked outside. I lost thirty pounds in six months, felt great doing it, and never once broke a sweat at a gym. More on this under the Parasites—Worms and Candida section later on in this chapter.

Gallstones—Cholesterol Deposits

At the end of the liver-gallbladder flush in the last chapter we finished the process by drinking the flavored bottle of magnesium citrate, followed by some water, and then went to sleep.

You don't want the toxins being released from the flush to be reabsorbed into your bloodstream, so the magnesium citrate effectively helps to move things quickly through your intestines. They will be flushed out the next day with the morning water and coffee enemas.

You may experience a need to use the bathroom during the night. If not, in the morning you will most likely have a bowel movement before your water enema. If you have a bowel movement before the water enema, that's fine, but you still need to do the water enema after the bowel movement. Some practitioners suggest putting a strainer in the toilet bowl before you go to bed so it's there before your first bowel movement that comes after your flush. The strainer will catch the *results* of your flush. If you have very hard gallstones, they would otherwise fall to the bottom of the toilet bowl, and you would never know it. So the strainer allows you to poke around in there to see what you can find.

While I slept the whole night, I did wake up a bit earlier than usual and had to use the bathroom right away. We were told this may happen and to expect the possibility. Even before the water enema I found still more surprises as the familiar ker-plunk and backsplash happened again. We didn't use strainers at HealthQuarters. This time I didn't need to fish too deep, as this surprise was floating! Yup, floating! We were told that our liver and gallbladder accumulates excessive and unprocessed cholesterol into varying sizes of *stones*. We were advised to look for pebble-to-pea-size or larger little floaters that may be covered in a brown or green fuzzy coating.

I had plenty to look at. They can be as small as dust bunnies and as large as the big shooter marble you used when you were a kid. You know—the big marble you balanced on your thumb nail and cradled up against your curled index finger before you gave it a push to knock out the smaller ones? (Does anyone besides me remember playing marbles?)

I didn't seem to have any hard gallstones, but I had plenty of the softer ones. Imagine how astonished I was when I saw some stones that measured one and a quarter inches long by an inch wide. Yes, I know the dimensions because not only did I fish those stones out of the toilet bowl, but I poked at them, too. I took them into the kitchen and sliced them up to see what else was in them, what their makeup was like. Yes, of course I used disposable paper towels and plates and a plastic knife. As I cut into one of the large green ones, I found it to be soft, very fatty in texture, and probably full of toxins. Yes, it was "show and tell" time again. I actually took some pictures from one of my monthly cleanses after I got home. I had to be a witness to people who wouldn't believe me otherwise.

I'm laughing so hard right now at the look I see on your face as you read this, and I'm listening to the thoughts roaming around in your head. Is she nuts! I'm going to do what? Poke around in there to see what I can find? No way! I am not going to do that!

Yup, that's exactly what I'm going to ask you to do. I used to keep a batch of long, wooden, BBQ skewers in the bathroom just for this purpose. Poking was half the fun. I got to see the results of what I was doing, and it was extremely revealing. Hey, you need to see for yourself the progress you're making and confirm for yourself that, yes, this program is working.

These soft, stone-shaped deposits were the consistency of Play-Doh; you could cut right through them. Not only did I measure them, but better than that, I took pictures to prove it. See!

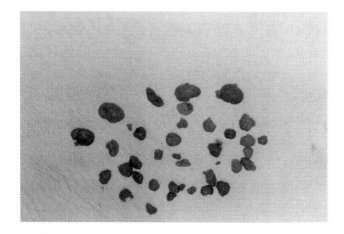

Dr. David Frahm at HealthQuarters suggested these were fatty cholesterol deposits consisting of unprocessed accumulated waste products in my liver and gallbladder because of the diet I was consuming. My diet was the culprit. My excessive food choices of junk food, dairy, fat, sugar, meat, white carbohydrates, and diet soda were over-taxing these organs. My liver and gallbladder just couldn't keep up with the diet. The *stones* were the consequence, the outcome, and a big reveal of my SAD diet. The stones plugged up my liver and gallbladder, preventing these organs from doing the filtering jobs they were designed to do

It took years of bad eating and lifestyle practices for me to get sick, so don't expect alternative options to get you well overnight. You will see improvement and it won't take long, but you will need to be patient and persistent.

I was truly beginning to understand the healing practices of alternative medicine. I saw the light at the end of the tunnel, and no, it wasn't a train. I was beginning to understand that my SAD diet and lifestyle were partly the cause of my cancer.

No wonder I got cancer. Except for my lungs, my heart, and my head it felt like none of my other organs were working the way they were supposed to work. My excessive SAD diet of almost fifty years caused me to get sick in a way I never thought I would. I thought I was doing the right thing, following the FDA-approved food pyramid. I learned how to cook and what foods to put on the table from my mother. No doctor would have suggested my choices were bad, except maybe to advise I exercise more and not eat as much at every meal. But they didn't say that either. What other organs were on their way to a malfunction that I didn't even know about yet.

Parasites—Worms and Candida

When I was at HealthQuarters, one of the Muscle Response Testing points indicated that I had parasites. I was told "we all do." What on earth was a parasite, and how did it get into my body? Where was it in my body, and how the heck do I get it out? All I knew about parasites was that dogs got tapeworms and other types of worms, and you gave them pills to take care of that problem a couple of times a year.

I learned that all produce, conventional and even organic fruits and vegetables, should be thoroughly washed, and in the case where there is a tough outer skin that can be scrubbed, scrub it. For everything else where scrubbing would otherwise destroy the fruit or vegetable, soak and gently rub wherever you can. You can use a solution of peroxide and water or white vinegar and water. There are many options on the Internet for a safe, economical, and effective vegetable wash. Pick one that feels right for you.

Why? When we purchase fresh fruits and vegetables they've just come from a farm, field of trees, low lying plant vegetation, and in the case of potatoes and other root vegetables, right out of the ground. They come to us usually with all kinds of oils, bacteria, pesticides, fertilizer residue, and wax coatings, especially if this produce is conventionally grown. So aren't these things washed off before we see them on the produce shelves and display cases? Yes, it has gone through a mild cleaning process, and I'm afraid to say that the water bath used to wash them is loaded with chlorine and fluoride, along with other chemicals from municipal water supplies.

Chlorine and fluoride are, of course, chemicals that we shouldn't be consuming under any circumstances, and we all know we drink a ton of it if we drink tap water. Yet still, by the time our produce is purchased by us, it's traveled through several processes. It's been picked, cleaned, packaged, shipped, unpacked and placed on the produce shelves. Many people have touched these fruits and veggies along the way. I'm not saying care isn't taken by the humans involved in this process, but parasites can come in from a variety of places and in a variety of ways that have nothing to do with human handling.

For instance, how many times do you buy a bunch of bananas, take them home, sit them on the counter, or place them on your banana hanger, and in a couple of days you have fruit flies taking over your kitchen? Where did these little buggers come from? The bananas looked clean and free of insects, right? Fruit flies leave little larvae all over fruits, and it's near impossible to be certain they won't be hatching unless we scrub everything we can and at least wash or soak everything else. You may say, "But I'm only going to eat what's inside the banana, not the skin, so why do I have to wash them before I eat them?" Simple. First, because you don't want those fruit flies doing acrobatics in your kitchen or laying eggs for further breeding somewhere else on an orange or mango you've just put in your fresh fruit basket on your counter. Second, and more important, when you go to peel the banana you're touching the outside skin, then throw the skin away, and then use your hands to eat the fruit inside. If there are any parasite eggs on the skin while you're peeling the banana, they can end up on your fingers, then in your mouth, and then ultimately take up residence in your intestines or somewhere else in your body.

Also, if you don't wash harder produce like melons, apples, and oranges, the knife you may use to cut them could contaminate the fruit as it cuts through the outer layer of unwashed skin and onto the meat of the fruit. You then put this into your mouth, and who knows where those little critters can become a not-so-welcome guest in your body?

You may also ask, doesn't the hydrochloric acid in my stomach take care of killing the parasites? Maybe yes, maybe no. As our SAD destroys our immune system and overall general health, many of our internal systems are just plain tired or have stopped working at peak efficiency. The production of hydrochloric acid could be one of your systems in disrepair. Some parasites have been around for thousands of years and have become resistant to all kinds of chemicals we otherwise think would kill them. Remember the cockroach? That bug just keeps getting bigger and bigger every year and more resistant to chemicals designed to eliminate it. It's similar to the millions of dollars' worth of antibiotics being doled out every time someone gets an infection and the doctor rushes to kill it off with the newest, latest, greatest version of antibiotics. Well, over time our bodies have become resistant to antibiotics. Our immune systems have lost their natural ability to kill off bacteria and viruses. Immune system failure is the reason we get sick or diseased in the first place.

So, anyway, here I am testing positive for parasites. I began taking a supplement called Para-Cleanse twice a day. Para-Cleanse is a supplement program whereby you take a packet of six pills two times a day, morning and evening, for ten days. The six pills collectively have the following ingredients, not in any particular order: paw paw cell-reg, pumpkin seeds, black walnut hulls, cascara sagrada bark, violet leaf, chamomile flowers, mullein leaves, marshmallow root and slippery elm bark, black walnut ATC concentrate, two species of Artemisia, wormwood and mugwort, elecampane root, clove flower buds, garlic bulb root, ginger root, spearmint herb, and turmeric root. All the ingredients were from some plant occurring in nature, many of which I had never heard of and knew nothing about. I felt like I was going to be living in the woods on nuts, seeds, and berries for the rest of my life. Little did I know how healing all these things were going to be without any side effects.

You take this ten-day supply twice a day, then stop for ten days, then take another ten day supply, then stop for ten more days, and then take one last round for ten more days. The Para-Cleanse kills only active adult parasites, not their eggs. So you give the little buggers in larvae stage time to hatch and then kill them off during the second and third ten-day cycles. Hopefully during the first ten days off after the eggs hatch the new little buggers haven't reached adulthood yet, so they haven't had time to make any whoopee and deposit more larvae on your intestinal walls. But just to be sure, it's recommended you do the last round. This cleanse is recommended twice a year.

Worms and Candida Forms of Parasites

Several times before the eight-day program at HealthQuarters was over, but after the impacted fecal-matter surprise, I had a few more unexpected *ker-plunks* with the first morning enema. These were large, tangled clumps of what looked like a bunch of light tan-colored rubber bands all balled up in a fist-size bundle. Were these worms or candida? I found pictures of what looked like tapeworms on the Internet that were very similar to what I saw in the toilet bowl. I wasn't sure what it was, except to know it was another wake-up call. I wasn't about to engage in fish, poke, and play again. This was just too disgusting, more so than the impacted fecal matter and the gall stones, which were just dead food particles, I thought. The worms or candida, well, that looked like a bunch of live organisms that took up residence, and that was truly a disgusting thought, but there it was, undeniably so.

I guess I was both glad and discouraged at the same time: glad that I was seeing real results of what the body can do when given the right tools to heal, and discouraged that the solution was so simple and yet my team of medical doctors had no knowledge of this. Alternative medicine wasn't something they could practice. After all it doesn't take a doctoral degree in medicine to administer raw fruits, vegetables, and juices to heal people. Yet it does take a lot of training to understand how all the more unusual natural herbs and spices can affect a very positive outcome. That's where a naturopathic doctor comes in: a doctor who understands the power of plants.

Anyway, all these incredible healing results were showing themselves in just eight days. If I was getting this much healing from just eight days, imagine what I could do in a year. I was beginning to get really excited.

In addition to getting parasites from raw fruits and vegetables, you can also get them from undercooked meat, pork, fish, and chicken. If you continue to eat meat after reading this book, at least make sure it's 100 percent grass-fed, raised in open pastures, organically grown, and humanely cared for and processed. In the case of fish, be sure it's wild and not conventionally farm-raised. There are massive amount of pesticides, herbicides, growth hormones, and antibiotics used in mass farming of pasture animals or farm-raised fish. In the case of dairy farming, the hormones injected into the animals are for the purpose of increasing milk production and in beef cattle to make them larger. Larger animals, larger yields, larger profits—follow the money. Our immune systems are already overtaxed. Purchase meat, pork, fish, and chicken from reputable organic farmers and resellers who care about what they grow, how it affects our ecosystem, and most importantly, how it affects you, the consumer.

Healing

When the parasites are gone, what happens to the tear in the intestinal lining? Quite simply, it heals, because at the same time you're doing this cleanse, you're also giving your body living food that it can use to heal itself. It's just like when you cut your finger. The healing nature of your body closes the wound, and you heal. The same thing happens on the inside. You're giving your body living food, nutrition in the purest form, dense with nutrients and enzymes. Freshly juiced apple and carrot juice and a product called Ultra Clear Plus from Metagenics also helped to detox and support my liver and gallbladder functions during the fast at HealthQuarters.

Charlotte Gerson is the founder of the Gerson Institute, which is located in San Diego, California. Dr. Max Gerson, Charlotte's father, developed the Gerson Therapy which is a non-invasive, alternative treatment for many chronic degenerative diseases, including cancer. Charlotte Gerson has said that when your body is healing from one thing, it quite naturally heals from everything. You can't just heal from one thing when you're giving your body what it needs to live. (Gerson 2013)

For the last sixty-plus years the climate of our food supply has been disintegrating. We've been mired in manufactured food and highly addictive food additives that are meant to create robotic eating machines of the human population with both serious and deadly consequences.

"Americans are the least healthy people among the world's developed nations (Japan, Australia, Germany, Canada, France, England etc.) In Fact there are even undeveloped nations that have healthier populations." (Brasscheck 2009)

"Healthcare spending in the U.S. is higher than that of most other developed nations-totaling roughly $7,290 per person – but the added costs have not translated into better care or quality of life." (Natural News.com "Higher US drug spending has not improved health" 2013)

Many processed food producers have contributed in making the United States stand out among the major industrialized nations because our health care costs are rising and there is no evidence of improved health. In fact the reverse is true. Doctors are prescribing more prescription drugs and we are being poisoned by them. This only serves to further weaken our immune systems, create more symptoms and side effects, which cause the doctors to prescribe yet more drugs.

Something is terribly wrong, and that is partly due to our falling for the incredibly good marketing efforts of the drug companies. They manage to convince us they have the answer for every single health problem we have: take one pill after another.

One commercial that drove me crazy was the one for restless-leg syndrome. Twitching in your legs is definitely a symptom of something. Do you need a drug to fix this problem? Maybe you need more exercise, maybe you need more magnesium, maybe you need more calcium or vitamin C, or maybe you just need to take a hot bath and relax.

We've become alienated from organic fresh fruits and vegetables and our kitchens. We've become overly dependent on the drug companies and their one-stop shopping campaign for everything needed to fix us; it's menacing and criminal. Ask any person who recovered from a grave disease or illness using alternatives, and they will tell you the same thing. Take responsibility for your own health, clean up your body, and you'll heal yourself from all disease and illness, not just one or the other.

Have you *ever* seen an overweight animal in their natural habitat? Animals don't get sick unless they get into something we humans have left behind as garbage for them to forage in or get trapped in.

Humans are not using what nature gives us to use as our food source, organic raw fruits and vegetables. We've been told we need meat and dairy by profiteers interested only in their quest to procure billions of dollars and to control their part of the world.

We're not idiots. We can make a choice to feed our bodies with food that's meant to nourish them, maintain our health, and allow us to live long, vibrant, wonderful lives.

In order to do this we have to get on the health bandwagon and out of the dependency program. You have to get out of your old story. Stop telling everyone how bad everything is in your life, comparing one doctor's opinion with another and sharing these stories with everyone you know.

Get a Vitamix high speed blender and a Champion Juicer or some other equivalent duo. These products are a bit on the expensive side compared to lower quality blenders and juicers, but what's your health worth to you? Do you just want to sit around and complain and be in your story or do you want to feel good? Do you want to play? Do you want to enjoy life? Gee, I hope so. *Then step out of your old story*, and step into a new one. Go beg, borrow or steal, well not really steal, these products and I can tell you you're days at the doctor's office will be gone with the wind. If you're healthy, you're having fun, following your passions and have fabulous things to do, you won't need your old story any more. So what are you waiting for? Go for it!

Observation

I was recently at a local hospital fitness center trying out a spinning class that a critical-care nurse friend of mine suggested. She loves spinning and had so much success getting her health back on track using spinning, among other exercises, that I thought I'd give it a try. She avoided knee surgery for a torn meniscus by losing eighty pounds—fifty pounds in the first year and thirty in the second year—by drastically changing her diet and undergoing a strict, self-imposed, regimented exercise plan, all on her own. Even she would not go under the knife to solve a health problem like this. She was too close to the profession and knew the problems that could occur with surgery, anesthesia, and drugs.

As I was leaving spinning class (not for me), I saw a man leaving the hospital supported by canes, two of them, one in each hand. He was seriously overweight, with legs that looked like tree trunks. There were wounds on his legs from the knee down that looked like they were never going to heal. I'm not being judgmental of this man, but there is something seriously wrong with that picture. We were not meant to live that kind of life. If you're healthy and you cut yourself, you heal and you heal quickly. Why is it there are so many critical wound-care healing centers? These people, in my opinion, need a huge diet overhaul to get their immune systems back in running order.

Impacted Fecal Matter—Testimony of Someone Else's First Hand Experience

I had been giving presentations in the community where I lived for several months, and naturally one of my favorite topics was impacted fecal matter. No, not to poke fun at people and their diets, but when you have the evidence of sickness staring at you in the face from the toilet bowl like I did, well, there's no more turning back.

I was beginning to have some *impact*, no pun intended, on some of the residents who were coming to the meetings and learning about a raw food diet, how powerful a cleanse can be, and some of the results that could be expected.

One of the residents, impacted (there I go again) by the information, decided to embark upon a colon cleanse, on his own, mainly because of irregularity. Several days into the cleanse he started to experience more regular bowel movements and had a more normal feeling in his lower abdomen, less bloating. A few days later I received a phone call from him telling me that he had been using a colon cleanse product for a few days and that he didn't feel well. He was sick to his stomach and feeling nauseous, lethargic, and tired. I said all those things are normal and positive side effects from a cleanse. They're signs the cleanse is working. The body is going through some radical detoxification and healing processes, and these side effects are related to the toxins being released from various parts of the body, particularly the colon. The toxins are causing these symptoms by traveling through the bloodstream before they have a chance to be released through more frequent bowel movements.

A couple more days went by, and he called me again, this time frantic and worried that something terrible was happening to him because he was really feeling quite ill—the same symptoms, but worse. Another friend of his suggested he go to a doctor or the emergency room, and that was certainly a choice he could have made.

On the same phone call he asked me if he was going to die (he felt that sick). He was very worried and sickened by what he saw in the toilet bowl. "I was freaked out," he said. He then proceeded to tell me that he had just passed this long chain of black chunky gunk through a bowel movement and was shocked to see so much of it in the toilet bowl.

"Dark, ugly fecal matter...Not me! Never could something so ugly possibly be in me," he said.

Needless to say, I was rejoicing and ecstatic for him. I praised him for having the courage to take on the challenge of a colon cleanse. This was just his first step in the process of cleaning out his body from years of eating the Standard American Diet, also known in some circles as *goo and glue*, resulting in the internal build up and release of this *dark, ugly fecal matter in the toilet bowl*.

He certainly could have gone to the doctor or the emergency room; however, he chose not to go. Each person is different and may experience a different set of circumstances. After a few more days he began to feel much better, and as he introduced more raw foods into his daily diet, he proceeded to lose thirty-five pounds. As a result of his revised diet and lifestyle, he no longer needed afternoon naps, had more energy, and looked fantastic.

More proof of the overall need for this kind of cleanse comes in an excerpt from *Tissue Cleansing Through Bowel Management* by Dr. Bernard Jensen, DC, Ph.D.: "The heavy mucus coating in the colon thickens and becomes a host of putrefaction. The blood capillaries to the colon begin to pick up the toxins, poisons and noxious debris as it seeps through the bowel wall. All tissues and organs of the body are now taking on toxic substances. Here is the beginning of true autointoxication on a physiological level." (Jensen 1981, 23) He goes on to say that: "One autopsy revealed a colon to be 9 inches in diameter with a passage through it no larger than a pencil! The rest was caked up layer upon layer of encrusted fecal material. This accumulation can have the consistency of truck tire rubber." (Jensen 1981, 27) This truck tire rubber is similar to what my friend experienced above. Dr. Jensen's book contains some incredible pictures of our digestive system which focus on the bowel and what it looks like when various diseases set in. He was an amazing researcher and health advocate.

There you have it from an expert in the field, my testimony, and that of a friend who experienced the effects of bowel cleanse. Do you need more convincing?

Symptoms of Detoxification

When and if you choose to embark on any part of a detoxification program, whether it's a colon cleanse, a juice fast, or anything else in between, please do so under the care of an alternative-care professional trained to guide you along the way, especially if this is your first attempt. You may experience many unpleasant side effects like fuzzy thinking, blurred vision, headache, lethargy, dizziness, grogginess, and having no desire for the usual things like coffee, alcohol, or sugar. These symptoms usually begin to show themselves within the first two or three days after the start of your cleanse. Try to have as much free time as possible before, during and after your cleanse, and be easy with yourself. Let your body perform the amazing things it can do—repair, regenerate and heal itself.

As was mentioned above with my friend who went through many of these symptoms, it can be a bit scary, especially if you experience the visual results that he did. You will realize how powerful detoxing is and begin to understand how infested your organs were with toxic buildup. I suggest to you, in spite of all of those symptoms, you will feel revived, renewed, and resurrected! You will feel overwhelmed with certainty and clarity that you have the power, with the right tools, to manage your own health.

Chapter Summary

You've been living a certain way for years, thinking all you need to do is take a pill when something happens. It's just not that simple, and besides, that pill just adds more toxicity to your already overtaxed immune system and it comes with so many side effects. Prescription drugs can also reduce or deplete your body from vitamin and mineral stores and continue to weaken your immune system. Is that what you really want? If so, as I said in the first chapter, go ahead, but that choice doesn't paint a very lively picture. This book is for people who want to make a life out of living. Consider this a serious and sobering wake-up call.

I became a lifelong alternative-medicine convert. I love my new lifestyle, way of healing, and belief system—completely. I became dedicated to sharing all the healing practices I learned that are steeped in the traditions of our forefathers and mothers. Let food be your medicine and medicine be your food. *First do no harm.* This is the way medicine is supposed to look—easy, without compromising side effects that could be worse than the disease itself.

I gave myself cancer, yes, indeed I did, and *I can take it away.* I gave myself cancer by by making low quality *food choices* and I took it away by making high quality *food choices.*

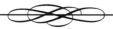

CHAPTER 9

Stress—Emotional, Spiritual, and Physical—and Detoxing Tools

ARE YOU HERE READING THIS book because you already have a disease or just because you want to improve your present state of health? Either way, you can eat all the raw food, drink the purest water, and breathe the freshest air, but without extinguishing negative, stressful feelings in all areas of your life, about yourself and others, or at least, learning how to better deal with these stressors, there's a good chance all the other great things you're doing won't work by themselves.

Stress kills, no matter what the form. Diseased thoughts, feelings, and emotions create physical illness in various parts of your body. Think of your cells as if each one were a separate muscle. That would be around 70 trillion muscles, as that is the approximate number of cells in your body. When you get agitated, angry, or wired mentally, emotionally, or physically what happens to your muscles? They tense up. When they tense up, blood flow is restricted. When blood flow is restricted, it creates these inflamed, knotted areas in those muscles and prevents necessary oxygen and nutrients from reaching their destinations.

If you've ever had a massage to help relieve stress related to tension from overworked muscles, a strain, or sprain, then you know a massage can restore the energy flow in that area of your body and how much better you feel after the massage. You're completely relaxed, for a while—until you go about your routine daily life and *stuff* happens to make you tense and uptight all over again.

The same thing happens to every cell in your body. Each cell is a living organism with a nucleus, a heart center, similar to your heart, and a heartbeat. Learning how to deal with stress is critical in overcoming disease. Even though you may be employing all the other solutions, without letting go of fear, anger, resentment, judgment, and other negative emotions you may never get well and stay that way. When you face a challenge of any kind—at work, at home, at play, or with your family—recognize the benefit it brought you. We all grow from contrast, and stress is just another form of being faced with something we don't want so we can focus on a better alternative, something we do want. Let go of the anger, quickly. Let it go and move on. If you dwell on any negative emotion long enough, it will eat you alive. Or, it can build you up and make you stronger. It's all in the perception of it.

What Does Stress Have to Do with Getting Cancer?

You might wonder what stress has to do with one woman's breast cancer recovery using alternatives. It's well known that cancer cells are ever-present in our body, and a healthy immune system keeps them from becoming anything more than a nuisance for the body to deal with on a daily basis—unless our diet and lifestyle tip the scales so off balance that cancer cells go unchecked, multiply, and actually do become a tumor growth. Cancer cells can begin to multiply and grow up to ten years before the actual discovery of a tumor large enough to be felt or seen on a mammogram or in X-rays.

Emotional stress is just now seriously being considered to have more significance in the cause of various diseases and illness than ever before. You can see references all over the Internet: "How Stress Causes Heart Disease," "Emotional Stress and Crohn's Disease - How They Relate," "Stress, Worry, and Anxiety," "Stress Linked to Cancer." There are hundreds.

Then there is physical stress—the kind that taxes the body in various other ways, from eating a poor diet, to feeling like the only way you can stay healthy is by running your legs off at a marathon pace and beating up on your muscles, joints, and bones, to pumping iron until your body is rock hard or doing other abusive physical exercise. Be gentle on yourself. To produce a healthy body you don't need to exhaust yourself, your schedule, or your time away from family, friends, or other activities you enjoy. And no, you probably won't be rock hard with this gentle approach, but you will not be physically stressed either.

Yoga, 5 Kriyas for Activating Kundalini, walking, and rebounding are just a few simple, no-impact types of exercises that will get you where you want to go, into a healthy physical body. If you want to run marathons or compete in the Olympics, that's a choice you make knowing both the positive and negative long-term consequences. Look at football players. They experience very short-lived professional careers because of the excessive physical abuse their bodies undergo in the short time they play. By the time they're thirty they're all used up. Make sense of your physical fitness plan. Don't overdo it; you don't have to. No pain, no gain? I don't believe that for a second.

Stress of every kind is hard on your body.

Emotional Detoxing

Emotional detoxing is getting rid of old patterns of living that no longer serve you. It's jumping to a new level of awareness. It's moving your energy to a higher place. Very simply, it's getting rid of your unresolved or repressed anger, grudges, bitterness, tension, control, envy, jealousy, hatred, judgment, and anything else that ties you up in knots. It's about making peace—first and foremost with you, then others, and then accepting and allowing all of it.

Are you unhappy with you? Are you unhappy about any certain aspect of yourself, your physical or emotional state? Are you holding any grudges against your spouse, your kids, your brother, your sister, your co-workers, or your parents? After all, your parents made you this emotional mess, right?

It's their fault you're in this horrible place, wherever that may be. You can blame them, the media, your politics, the way the world is, your friends, your teachers, or anyone else you want.

However, all that negative thinking is part of how you may have acquired this diseased state to begin with; get rid of it! It's just not serving you any longer. Your parents gave you life, food, shelter, and safety. After that, the rest of your life is what you made it through your own choices and decisions, and your life will be what you make it going forward. It's all up to you, whether you believe it or not. You're in charge of making choices; you always have been; you always will be. You're in charge of taking responsibility for your actions, all of them. You're in charge of the consequences of literally everything in your life, good and bad!

I believe that part of the reason we may get illness and disease is because we get stuck in our story about why and how things have happened in our lives. Are you blaming everyone in your life for where and what you are right now? *Get off that soapbox!* It's just bringing you deeper and deeper into an intense, unfathomable abyss, and unless you change your attitude, you're never going to get out of it. You put yourself in there, and you have this horrible story about all the details of your life. You're certainly entitled to your story, and you're entitled to stick with your story for as long as you want. But I can tell you first hand that it's no longer serving you and it never did. In fact, these tied-up fears and emotions could very well be the reason for your sickness, or diseased body.

When you come across a person on the street who just simply smiles at you, for no good reason, just because they're a happy person, don't you smile back at them? You may be miserable in your story, but today you meet a happy person who smiles at you. Doesn't it feel good to see that smile and smile back? The wrinkles on your forehead lift and disappear too! Suddenly, for a moment, you're in a good place. What would happen if you could feel this way every moment of every day? Try initiating a smile sometime, for no good reason. Doesn't just the thought of that put you into a better place? When you put a whole lot of those smiles together with good thoughts and feelings, it becomes a string of benefits to your immune system that you just can't live without.

I just want you to know that I love you—yes you—the person holding this book in their hands, and I don't even know you personally. I love you, just because I know that I am you, and you are me. Feel that energy!

Do this right now. Go to a mirror. Look deep into the center of your eyes and say, "I love you!" Don't be timid about this. Yell it out loud, and feel it in your heart and in your soul. *I love you!* Then, at the same time, smile as you say this again. Now wrap your arms around yourself, smile, look into the mirror, and say, "I love you" again.

This little gesture of loving yourself and smiling can be the beginning of getting out of your old story and into a new and better story. I would like you to smile, for as long as you can, for no other reason than just because it feels good. As you are showering, making your morning breakfast, changing the oil in your car, driving to work, walking around the grocery store. Smile! Gee, that feels good, doesn't it, and it can't help but put you in a good mood. Try wearing a smile for as long as you can and see what it does for your disposition and those around you. You'll start to make other people smile and what could be more fun than to watch their reactions to a smile? You're smiling on your way to loving yourself and to a happy place you may not have known before. You can't help but think happy thoughts. You can't help but start to feel better. Who cares what other people may think when they see you smile and no one else is around? Saying I love you and smiling are two of the biggest things you can do to get over your old story and begin a healing. Your cells love you right back for it. As you do these things you can't help but feel great. *Yes, today is the first day of the rest of your life.*

The first thing you're going to do is learn to love yourself, unconditionally, warts and all. The moles on your nose, the hair growing out of your ears (by the way, they make clippers for that), your saggy butt or boobs, your big belly, your thick thighs, your ample ankles, your balding head, your fat feet (that's my problem, among others)—whatever it is you feel are your worst characteristics. Love each and every one of them.

I don't say this lightly. Do you understand how infectious a bad attitude is—a grumpy face, someone constantly complaining, who never finds a good thing to say about anyone or anything? I'm talking about it being infectious to you, and if you start to become like this person you will infect people around you, too, including your family and friends. You're creating an illness or disease and putrefaction so deeply inside you that the consequences can be quite literally, unimaginable. Besides all that, these attitudes show themselves on your face; as in the dulled sparkle of your eyes, the wrinkles on your forehead, or the frown on your lips. You can look alive and loving or depressed and fearful. It's your choice. Everyone wears their emotions and most of it shows up on your face, and in your body language.

I'm sure you've been around both types of people before, and I hope you're not one of the grumpy ones. If you are, take a serious look at what this is doing to your body, mind, and spirit. My guess is that it's doing nothing but putting you in a bad mood every day and perhaps creating more negative relationships than positive ones.

I've had the pleasure of meeting a lot of wonderful people, but I've also encountered some who were so negative I couldn't wait to get out of their presence. I wanted to run hard and fast in the opposite direction. I want no part of these people or the energy created by them. It's not so hard to believe that positive and happy people also seem to be healthier than those who have a pessimistic view of the world. They may not be problem free, but how they handle day-to-day activities goes a long way toward how they project themselves to others and to themselves.

Since I gave myself an attitude adjustment years ago, all I want to do is be close to people who are uplifting and say wonderful things about their life, no matter what may be going wrong in their world. There is nothing going on in our lives that we don't somehow invite in through our thoughts, which become our feelings, and those feelings eventually manifest as our reality.

So today, start your new story. Decide what it is you want from life— your emotional side, your spiritual side, your mental side, and your physical side. Start your new story. You're the creator of it, only you.

I know it's easy for me to say *start your new story today,* but how? I'm going to suggest some things a little later on that may seem foreign to you, but they work. Open the doors of your life, take the top off the box, step out and look at things with a new pair of eyes. If you're just settling, go for something you really want, elevate your life and your mood. What have you got to lose? If you're already sick and miserable, you've got nowhere to go, but up!

My Life and Stress

Growing up, I encountered an incredible number of stressful situations. I grew up in a very modest, camp-style home that I had to walk into through many inches of snow every night in the middle of the winter because the roads were private and unplowed. We towed our groceries in behind us on a toboggan. My bedroom had unfinished plywood floors that could give me splinters. I went to sleep watching light beams reflecting from walls covered with Owens Corning aluminum-faced insulation in between two by four inch studded walls, because they were unfinished too.

My father was not there emotionally for me, drank excessively, gambled, and ran around with other women. I so wanted to feel his love and never did. My mother, next to the youngest of nineteen children, knew very little of supporting her own children in their emotional growth, so I received no feelings of love from her either. An initially very happy and fulfilling marriage became difficult with the added responsibility of parenthood. A brilliant child with a mind of his own gave us challenges for which we were unprepared. I was addicted to an outdated religious belief system as a Roman Catholic and was scared to death of the God I was introduced to growing up, right up until I was diagnosed with breast cancer at fifty years of age. I chose to be wrapped up in career that drained me, emotionally and physically, every day to the point I had little energy left to give my family or my friends. All this and more created a fertile ground for cancer growth.

I was angry at my parents uninvolved way of nurturing, for growing up in such a depressed physical environment, having a roller coaster of a marriage, difficulties in parenting, you name it, I was mad at it. I buried myself in my work hoping to find some sort of relief or satisfaction that would melt away the pain I was hiding from and didn't even know was there.

I won't blame my upbringing, my parents, or anyone else for my life and all that it brought me, good and bad. As adults we all have the freedom of choice, to change our experience if we don't like where we are. What happens when we're young goes a long way to mold and set the stage for who and what we become as adults, or so we think. Imagine how our life could be different if we were given unconditional love and support as a child growing up. I don't feel I got much, if any, of that, yet I did manage to make some good choices and became a contributing member of conventional society instead of one who drew from the system. You can change, right now. All you need is the will and desire to become that person you want to be.

Cancer and Anger

I have to share the story of a very close friend that speaks to this situation. A male friend of mine had been diagnosed with cancer. After the initial diagnosis he chose to use alternatives to care for his body and see if this could restore his health. Alternatives worked for a while, a couple of years, in fact. However, the cancer returned, and he ultimately died after resorting to traditional treatments like chemotherapy, radiation, and additional surgery.

The problem, as I see it, was not his choice of treatment the first time around, but failing to see, believe, and utilize the fourth element of healing, which is letting go of bottled up negative emotions and stress. You simply must lose the fear, the judgment, the criticism, and the anger; lose all those negative feelings about everybody and everything, yourself included.

You know what they are because you know what and who pushes your buttons to make you upset. Because I knew this person so well, I knew much of the family history and stories associated with the anger and resentment he felt. His heart ached for family peace and for things he could not control. Yet he still wanted to manipulate the lives of his children and their interaction with each other.

He became a victim of self-imposed adverse circumstances. He ultimately did give up control with his death. Is that what you want for your life? You've heard the phrase about someone who is very frugal with money—"You can't take it with you"? Well, this guy did take his emotions and his disease with him, to the grave. His expiration date was up, but it was self-imposed.

What was so powerful in this man's life that he couldn't give up—even when it might cause his death? The ego is a righteous inflation of pride and makes us all victims of our own painful and pitiful thinking. What makes us want to be right so much that we choose death over life? Instead of just letting these emotions go and realizing the only person he had control over was himself, he just became an angry person and, in my opinion, died because of it. Anger, a new, maybe not so new, cause of death!

Do I have any proof of this? No. Do I need any? No! Why? Because I used to be an angry person, too. I used to let my ego and anger rule. When I finally realized the only person I had control over was me, I let everything else go. However, all that came after my cancer diagnosis.

The consequence of letting go was an overwhelming, joyous feeling of freedom that continues to this day. This freedom to love myself and others unconditionally supplies me with enough energy and positive feelings to jettison me into each and every new moment of *now*. *Now*: that's all there is. Right now, not yesterday, not tomorrow, just right now. How you treat yourself and others in this one single moment of time will determine your health as much as all the other things I've already mentioned. When you learn to respect everyone for their gifts and what you perceive to be their problems, you can't help but recognize the always, ever-present abundance of love and joy that surrounds you and that is you.

That, my dear friends, is where it all starts. Love yourself first, and then you can't help but love everyone else. You will radiate such positive energy that the cells in your body will receive the organic raw food and juices, the clean air, the pure water, with such love and positive intention that they will help you create the new you, a surviving, thriving, joyous, and vibrant new you!

Then you will know that no one can hurt you, not even your kids, who won't listen to the wisdom of your years or take advantage of your life experience. You will be free from any feeling of need to push them. They are adults now, they can choose to do, say, be, or act in any way they choose for themselves. Knowing they chose for themselves frees you. Do you understand just how powerful this is? *You are free* of responsibility for anyone, except yourself.

I know this is true because all alternative therapies I've read suggest many different ways to let go of control and focus only on love.

Don Miguel Ruiz, author of *The Four Agreements* and now, in collaboration with his son Don Jose Ruiz, co-author of *The Fifth Agreement: A Practical Guide to Self Mastery* talks about these precise things and how to apply these agreements so you can obtain eternal happiness right here and now. (Ruiz 1997) (Ruiz, Ruiz and Mills 2010)

Doctor's Ego

I have to share this story here because *I allowed it* to bring me to such a place of anger and become so filled with rage, I just wanted to scream.

I was trying to wrap up my doctors appointments in New York before heading back to Florida for the winter, and one of my last visits was to Dr. Christine. I wanted a female medical doctor who was paying attention to alternatives, and she was recommended by a friend, so I became her patient. She was my primary-care physician, and since she was a family practitioner it was easy to get multiple things accomplished with just one visit.

After I brought her up to speed about my breast-cancer history, she was insistent that I pay a visit to her favorite oncologist, one who she highly recommended, so that in the event I had a recurrence, I would already have established a relationship with him. This was a different oncologist from the one I saw with my original breast-cancer diagnosis.

My heart wasn't really into going to see another doctor, especially an oncologist, who I didn't think I would ever need. And what oncologist wanted to interview a *prospective* cancer patient? I was a *cured* ex-cancer patient. He was accustomed to administering to sick people. I was beyond healthy. However, I put my reservations aside, made the appointment, and sent out various letters of request to all the other doctors who previously treated me in order to release my medical records to him. He would need to review my case history before my appointment.

He came into the exam room, had my very thin folder in his hands, and asked, "So, Linda, what can I do for you?" I shared with him how disappointed I was that our current medical system did not allow alternative doctors to request various scans and other noninvasive tests on behalf of their patients. These tests could help monitor the healing progress of cancer patients who chose to use alternative methods for their treatment plan. I also shared my disappointment that alternative doctor visits and tests were not on the approved and covered expense list of many health-insurance companies. This, of course, meant people who chose alternatives would have to pay for these tests directly, out of their own pockets. One of these tests, which I did have, was called an AMAS test. That stands for Anti-malignin Antibody in Serum test, which measures cancer-cell activity in the blood. I went to Boston for that test because the blood had to be fresh and tested right away. This and other tests, like ultrasounds and MRI's, a naturopathic doctor or alternative health-care provider cannot order.

I mentioned to the oncologist that if I did actually get a cancer recurrence I would probably choose to do the same thing over again, use alternatives. I mentioned that I would like to use his services to write prescriptions for various tests and scans to monitor my alternative progress.

He looked me square in the eyes and said, "Well, Linda, that wouldn't be very rewarding for me now, would it?"

I wanted to slap him for his arrogance. Rewarding for him? You have to be kidding me. To think a doctor is in the profession of making people well to serve his own ego is pitiful, deplorable, and just plain reprehensible. Needless to say, we were done, kaput, finished as they say. This is one of the reasons the health care system is really sick—doctors who get into the business to serve their own egos and don't give a real rip about their patients' state of health. (Of course I know I'm generalizing here and know not all doctors are that self serving.)

I left his office and stopped at the checkout to pay my co-pay. The
female attendant behind the desk began to ask me all kinds of questions
about what tests I needed to have done. I said I don't need any tests.

She then asked, "Why are you here?"

I said I was hoping to find a traditional doctor who would be willing
to work with a prospective cancer patient who wanted to use alternatives
to regain her health, if and when the time came.

She asked sheepishly under her breath, "Did you find one?"

I shook my head no, paid my co-pay, left, and never went back. She
seemed quite sympathetic in her visual responses.

So it seems what we have here is a health-care system set up to support
some doctors' self-serving egos in the medical profession. The approach
seems to be, if you don't take my caustic and harmful treatments, I don't
want to be your doctor. My words, not his, but you can see the injured nature
of this system when the value of a doctor's ego outweighs the good of the
patient. There is room in the health-care system for both modalities, and I
know there are more of these integrative and complimentary approaches
now beginning to work together, even though many of the alternative
options are still not covered by health insurance.

The health-care system is badly broken. The delivery and cost of
treating my cancer could have easily been in excess of $100,000 with
traditional treatments and western allopathic methods. We actually spent
around $14,000 that first year for supplements and various other alternative
health-care professionals' office visit fees, lab tests, and such that were
not covered by our insurance. Subsequent years' expenses were less as I
regained my health and relied more on organic food and less on vitamin
and mineral supplements to keep my restored immune system strong.

My alternative choice would have cost so much less for my health-
insurance company to cover that it's almost inconceivable they don't
consider alternative-services payable claims. Yes, I had the ability to claim
my medical expenses over the allowable limit on my tax return, but why
aren't all medical expenses deductible to begin with, and why can't these
expenses just be paid by health-insurance companies?

I would have been willing to sign all kinds of waivers claiming I would not file a lawsuit in the event of an unsatisfactory outcome with alternative options in place of traditional ones. I would have signed a waiver for every technician, doctor, hospital, and clinic that was involved in my care in any way. I did have a favorable outcome without traditional medical treatments. A person's choice of treatment should be the patient's choice, not a medical dictate or cost prohibitive.

This story is meant to show you just how mad and angry I was. It took me a long time to let go of this anger. It took me years, not just a few days, weeks, or months. However, I had to let it go. I had to recognize these doctors went through a lot of education, specialty training, and expense to learn how to apply all these deadly treatments of chemical cocktails, radical radiation, and surgery. I did let it go. Selfishly, I let it go because my own health was at stake, and I wasn't about to let some inconsiderate, egotistical, poor excuse for a doctor ruin my life. And in my heart I know not all doctors are driven by ego. So I made peace with it. A friend shared an ancient Hawaiian tradition of forgiveness and reconciliation called Ho'o pono pono. This little practice went a long way in helping me overcome this angry situation, among others.

Ho'o pono pono

You say, "I love you"; "I am sorry"; "Please forgive me"; and "Thank you." These four short phrases free you like nothing you've ever experienced before. It's a short yet very powerful method of releasing anger and judgment. I was the one who got angry regardless of the circumstances; I was the one who initiated the anger. No, you don't have to say this Ho'o pono pono prayer directly to or in front of the person you're asking forgiveness from. It can be said silently but with intention and most of all, sincerity. You do need to open yourself up, become vulnerable and transparent. Why would you want to be anything less?

Here's how it works. You say, "I love you." They are human beings and don't deserve at any level to be treated in whatever way you treated them. What you see in other people is generally a reflection of who you are. These things are in you or you wouldn't be experiencing them. So yes, you say "I love you," and as you do, you are saying this to yourself as well because we are all related. I am you, you are me, and we are one.

You say, "I'm sorry" for any hurt or harm you may have caused this person. This releases you from the negative reverberating effect this bad feeling had: in my case, not just on me and the doctor, but on everyone else who came into contact with that negative emotion in any way. Remember, emotions are vibrations that touch whatever comes into contact with them. Vibrations also reverberate throughout eternity and touch people, places, and things we don't even know about. My family and friends got an earful of my negative emotion around that particular incident for a very long time.

You say, "Please, forgive me" because you truly want the other person's forgiveness, and you want to forgive yourself for this negative experience. You want them to accept your apology graciously and genuinely. As you reach out and ask for forgiveness, you demonstrate your sincerity, and a healing begins.

You say, "Thank you" for *listening* and *feeling* this new vibration of love, kindness, and appreciation. You both then have grown, by learning to extend and accept forgiveness. Thank you for bringing this situation into my awareness and for the gift or gifts it brings. A new love vibration is set in motion and sent out to the universe.

Love heals, hate hurts! Let's make love a regular daily standard for everyone and everything, everywhere. You don't have to be in a romantic place of love with someone to tell them you love them, just love them as another human being. Many people I know get really confused about saying, "I love you," thinking that if they say those words someone will think they are romantically "in love" with them. You know the difference, so start saying "I love you" when you leave someone, when you end a telephone call, and as you sign off from e-mails and letters to your family and friends. Let us love one another and not be afraid to show it or say so.

I continued to apply Ho'o pono pono in all aspects of my life in areas where I had hurt someone or where someone hurt me. This practice works both if you are the one doing the hurting or the one who was hurt. This ancient Hawaiian tradition of Ho'o pono pono makes so much sense to me. The reason it's so powerful is because when you recognize that what you do to someone else, you actually do to yourself, you truly understand the meaning of forgiveness.

Ho'o pono pono helped me to heal the emotional scars I endured, or, shall I say, inflicted upon myself, from my negative feeling toward my father and mother to my relationships with other family members and friends. Again, the other person doesn't have to be present to hear this apology face-to-face for it to be effective. What you are doing is sending positive, compassionate, love vibrations out to replace the negative emotions you sent before. The old negative vibrations are transformed into love vibrations.

After you've released all this negative emotion, the cells in your body will reawaken and can then actually use all the other gifts you're sending their way, like organic raw food and pure water and air. It's a quadruple win! A guaranteed success!

Here's a wonderful YouTube version of this Ho'o pono pono song. It's just beautiful. (Depaula 2010)

Organ Crunchers

Research studies have identified that when negative toxic emotions are allowed to control a person's ongoing response to life, they can produce possible harmful disruptions to body chemistry.

Aggressive hostility activates the release of stress hormones that send the body into red alert—the *fight-or-flight response*. That's fine if you need to run for your life, but in today's world this rush is more consistently felt throughout the better part of a person's day, and even considered routine. Upset, other than in appropriate circumstances, is a recipe for a health disaster, not to mention other possible disastrous consequences.

Following is a partial list of various emotions and what organ may possibly be affected by that long-term unresolved poisonous emotion that you're carrying. The root of these associations is based on traditional Chinese medicine. (livestrong.com 2013)

- Anger, Bitterness, Resentment   Liver, Gallbladder
- Anxiety, Grief, Inflexible,
  Defensive   Lungs, Large Intestine
- Pensiveness, Melancholy   Spleen, Digestive System
- Fear, Disharmony, Terror   Kidneys, Involuntary Urination

You can see from this list what organ may be affected by any long-term acute, unresolved feeling or emotion. If you're experiencing fear or terror of anything, your kidneys may be affected. If you suffer from anger, bitterness, or resentment, your liver may be affected. Long-term unresolved negative emotions can ruin your health, your work, and your relationships.

Some research has indicated that the leading cause of death in adults over sixty five is disease related to unresolved hurt, which is equivalent to stress. This statement takes me back to my male friend who tried alternatives, recovered for a couple of years, and then died anyway. My recollection of his situation was one of massive, unresolved family conflict at every turn, coming on like machine-gun fire from all directions and his inability to deal with it, let it go, and just focus on himself.

Fear

Fear is paralyzing, crippling, handicapping, and it's a wake-up call for you to examine what's really going on in every area your life. Fear just makes your soul hurt and inhibits your mental, emotional, and spiritual growth and perhaps the physical nature of who you are as well. What are *you* afraid of?

As I grew and let go of fear and allowed love to find a stronghold in my life, I became transparent. I cleaned the cobwebs off the ceiling, and I let pride and ego melt away, as much as I could on a daily basis. For each of us this will happen at different speeds. The quicker you can make it happen in your own life, the better it will be. Your experiences of the world around you will look and feel rewarding, whereas before they were restricting. It will be liberating. You will find a new sense of freedom that you never thought could or would be part of who you are. You will be emancipated from shackles that bind you. Judgment, criticism, and other people's views of you no longer matter because, once and for all, you now know who you are. It's the proverbial snowball rolling down the hill, and this time, it's such a lovely snowball!

I simply love being transparent now. The amount of love that has found its way into my heart is immeasurable. The ripples of love, the vibrations of love, the energies of love that you send out find their way back to you over and over again. I'm surrounded by happy and loving people, and I now truly enjoy the most incredible friends and community.

This does not happen easily, as we are surrounded by mass media telling us how to think, how to feel, what to buy, where to buy it, what we should look like, and if we don't do as they say, we won't be accepted. Accepted by whom? Them? Who are they but some big corporate conglomeration of self-serving big businesses? The only thing they're interested in is their bottom line, their net income. Do you want to be afraid of someone you don't even know, just because they may have more money or appear more powerful?

How about the centuries of fear instilled by various religious institutions for not doing the right thing? Doing the right thing, according to whom— church leaders, most of whom were power and money-hungry men who wanted to control their kingdoms in self-serving ways? Fear is a great motivator, and many rulers were extremely successful in building their empires using fear.

When these religious and business organizations got you attached to them emotionally and mentally from the time you were a child and you've grown with their philosophies into adulthood, well, now it's time for a spiritual detox. When you go through a lifetime of believing you have no control over your own thoughts or belief systems and you've been sold someone else's righteous ideas of what you and the world should look like, those are things many religious and political wars have been fought over. And we're still fighting them. So where's the progress?

You can let go of fear and let love in. The best part of realizing that love is a much better state to be in than fear is realizing that you have to love yourself first before you can love anyone or anything else.

Fear makes you a prisoner of your life and your soul. I beg you, please, try to find someone to talk with about working through and giving up your fears, no matter what they are.

Meditation

I didn't know what meditation was until I was diagnosed with cancer and went to HealthQuarters. I thought it was just some weird way of escaping reality. It is definitely an escape from reality, but it is healing and renewing at the same time. Meditation is unquestionably a getaway from things that bug you, irritate you, make your blood boil, and make the hair on the back of your neck stand at attention. Meditation is definitely one way to let go of whatever it is that's upsetting you so you can calm down and return to your daily routine feeling refreshed. Meditation isn't going to make your problems go away, but it will give you a better state of mind in which to deal with your problems.

Some people have this idea that you have to sit on a meditation pillow, with your legs crossed, sitting straight as a poker with your eyes closed, chanting *Ohm* with your thumb and middle fingers touching each other in the shape of a circle. Of course, if that appeals to you, great, but it's not the only way.

Meditation can be as simple as lying down on your bed and taking a rest for a few minutes. If you're working, go to the lounge, or to the bathroom if that's the only place you can go, and just *be* quiet for a few minutes. Stop the noise, the chatter, and the incoming and outgoing mental messages. Stop long enough to rest for a short time and let these thoughts just flow in and out very gently. I know this has been said and labored to death, but, focusing on your breathing works wonders to clear your mind. You forget everything else for just a few minutes.

There's a beautiful meditation that a friend, author and medium Suzanne Giesemann co-created with the most beautiful soul-elevating music from French composer Frederic Delarue. This meditation is just twelve minutes long and is a free download. I highly recommend you listen to this piece because it could create a critically needed time of peace that could be helpful in re-creating your day, and only twelve minutes away, anytime you want it. (Giesemann 2013)

Letting Go

Letting go! What does this mean, to let go of something? When people talk about letting go of something it's usually a thought that's created a negative stronghold in our head that we can't seem to stop thinking about. That just about sums it up for me. Years ago when I got really upset or angry at something, I remember being so tensed up about it that it would literally take me at least three days to get over it. Get over it? No, I didn't get over it. I just buried it in my head someplace for it to come up again at some future time. The thought was gone, but not forgotten.

Truly letting go of something means to think of it as a neutral event in my life. It happened, and everything that happens to you comes for a reason. To grow, to learn, to experience, to allow you to make choices, all kinds of choices, isn't life grand? If we become stagnant, what happens? We die. We emotionally die. There are times in my life when I certainly felt that way. I don't want to feel that way anymore, and while I've made great strides in letting go of things, I still work on it.

You no longer think of this problem as a reason to upset you. An event happened, that's all. It's all neutral. Why do we get angry at things that upset us to the point of having to let it go to begin with? Usually it's because something didn't go our way. Someone didn't do what we wanted or expected them to do. You let this person or situation ruin your day. Do you really want that to happen? I'm sure you've all been there at one time or another. If you haven't, you're very fortunate!

Years later, I've come to learn that letting go for me means releasing the negative energy and no longer lingering on the thought of it. If a circumstance comes into my awareness that's not pleasing, I either remove myself from the situation or start doing some deep breathing and refocus on something else. Deep breathing helps to oxygenate the body, as we've discussed previously, but it also causes us to release tension. Tension is usually what causes us to feel negative emotion, anyway. So deep breathing is a wonderful tool. The other thing I do, especially if it was a person who irritated me, is surround that person with love energy. How do you do this? I just imagine this person surrounded by beautiful white light and see this light penetrating into the very core of their body. This is incredibly healing for me, and I believe it's helpful to the other person as well.

We've all found ourselves in a heavy traffic jam or two at one time or another. What can you do to relieve the angst? Get angry, blow the horn, roll down the window, pound the steering wheel, shake your fist at someone and start yelling at people who can't do any more about it than you can. Take some deep breaths, put on some soothing music, be patient, relax, and wait. Take a little vacation while you're at it. Think of the most inviting vacation you can imagine, whether it's to a sunny, sandy beach or some snowy-white mountains for a ski trip or to an historic, old town with lots of shops and museums or to a wine-tasting tour through Italy. Wherever it is, go right there, in that very moment. You don't even have to close your eyes to do this. (I wouldn't recommend that anyway if you're in your car). Ahh! Now doesn't that feel better?

Most often when we're angry it's due to some judgment being assessed. If we didn't have judgment, we wouldn't become angry at anyone, or anything, at any time, for any reason. What a peaceful world I'm describing here, right? Well, you can have this world, but it will take a bit of adjusting.

There are many spiritual books, practices, and websites to begin your search. I've studied many of them, some more intensely than others, but all say practically the same thing. One I am particularly drawn to is Ester Hicks, a woman who connects with a consciousness field called Abraham that teaches a very basic lesson that's really hard for many of us to understand and more difficult to apply. It's called *get happy*. Yes, it's that simple, get happy. Stop trying to row your boat upstream against the current. Pull the oars inside the boat and let the boat float downstream. Let the energy of life and the universe take you where you need to go. How do you know where the boat will take you? You set your intentions and desires and focus on those things that will bring you the most joy, you get happy. Abraham's guidance helped me make sense of my spiritual, physical, mental and emotional sides to my life. Many helpful resources to begin your journey are available from the Abraham-Hicks website, books, dvd's, cd's, cruises, workshops and more. (abraham-hicks 2013)

Becoming a vibrational match is another Abraham teaching. If you want people, things, and circumstances that are currently not in your life, then you must become a vibrational match to those things in order to achieve the outcome of your desires. If you want to be around happy people, become a happy person; it is that simple. You can't expect to be living a miserable story and bring happy people into your life.

I'm going to take you back to my ballroom dancing experience again in order to explain what being a vibrational match means to me. When I first heard about Abraham's vortex of attraction, the escrow, and becoming a vibrational match to that which you seek, I was bewildered. What did this mean, and especially how did I apply it in my own life?

I've always wanted to be a ballroom dancer, not at a competitive level but just to dance. The romance and the unity of two people flowing and dancing together in harmony on the dance floor is something I am incredibly passionate about. The image still, as I share this, brings me to tears, to *feel* that oneness with another person in the magic of the dance as beautiful music plays, creates an exhilarating effect throughout every cell in my body. This desire was so strong it was unimaginable to me how I was going to express and accomplish this. I put my fears and reservations aside. I made some phone calls, signed up for some lessons, and here I am, fulfilling my passion. I am now in vibrational alignment with my desire. It's manifested, and it's here now for me to enjoy. You can't expect Prince Charming to come and sweep you off your feet if you don't become a princess, walk the walk, talk the talk, or dance the dance. You have to become what you desire.

Every one of you possesses a passion for something in your life. If you don't, you're already half dead. Get a life! Go find your passion and breathe it, do it, become it, live it! To get in alignment with my passion as a dancer was to feel my way into it, to know that I could, and the universe would then make the rest of it happen. When you're excited and feel great about something, you're halfway to your goal. Follow your heart!

I did follow my passion, twice. The first time I put myself into vibrational alignment was with my cancer diagnosis, and although it was a deliberate alignment, I didn't know the definition of what I was doing at the time. I had undeniable desire and commitment to the goal. That time I overcame cancer and got well using alternative solutions. It was simply putting the law of attraction and the power it holds to work. It was the desire to live in a vibrant, healthy body. Presto! Mission accomplished! The second time it was with an absolute knowing I needed to dance, specifically, to get involved with ballroom dancing.

Remember when we talked about the morning enema routine and how I would light a candle, put on some soft music, and sometimes I would meditate on being whole again? Sometimes I would put the vision of my body healing in the forefront of my mind and visualize my body returning to a complete state of wellness. I would watch as my cells, one by one, would return to a healthy state.

What I did was get into vibrational alignment with my desire. Seeing the results of my vision, before the manifestation, before the reality showed itself, was part of the process and so compelling. It was a dream that came true of nuclear proportions. It is that powerful!

You need to do your part to create the wellness you desire. Your part in overcoming your current physical condition is to *visualize* yourself in a complete state of wellness, believing it will happen, and doing things that are right for you that will bring that healing about.

When I first started down this spiritual path, I started reading books by Caroline Myss, Ph.D., Eckhart Tolle, Neale Donald Walsch, Esther Hicks, Gary Renard, Louise L. Hay, and Dr. Wayne Dyer, among others. Books like *A Course in Miracles* and *The Secret* were also real eye openers. The various perspectives I read about from these authors woke me up like a Polar Bear Club member jumping into a partly frozen snow-covered lake in the middle of winter. Brrrrrr! Those books got my attention. I was awake, or at least I was beginning to see the light, and it wasn't a train at the end of a tunnel. (Schucman 1976) (Byrne 2006)

The one thing that resonated throughout all of this material is that we are responsible for one thing and one thing only: ourselves. The choices we make every moment of every day create our lives. We own those choices. We can't blame other people for the way we behave, our thoughts, or our actions. We are in total control. No one else is, just us. Forget whatever programming you received growing up, especially if it was a major dose of fear-based religion. Just my opinion, but that's the worst kind. You can make new choices for new programming that truly serve who you are now and who you want to become.

I realized that I had a choice to make regarding my life. Did I want to live the way I wanted to live? Or, did I want to live according to someone else's *design plan* for life? I chose to write my own *design plan*, and I will decide what that plan will look like. I will be the creator of my own life. I chose to use alternative solutions to solve my cancer problem. Poof! No more cancer problem or health issues of any kind.

Am I going to be climbing Mount Everest anytime soon? No, but if I wanted to, I would train like hell to achieve it, and I would. That is desire. That is why Olympians push so hard and reach their goals. They have tremendous desire and visualize the results of their efforts during training even before the competition begins. I believed I was already cured even before it happened. I became an Olympic champion of my own health and so can you!

Support

If you're on the receiving end of what you perceive to be a lack of support, please try to understand and forgive what you think may be injustices done to you. Another's journey is their journey, and it's very hard for anyone to know what's gone on in the background, even if it's your own family. Stress, in the form of a major illness, brings out character traits you never saw before in people you think you knew very well. Sometimes you just don't, until a stressful situation presents itself.

If you're unable to support a loved one going through a difficult time or are critical and can't find love in your heart to affirm and sustain them because of your own inner conflict with the direction they chose, please, please, please try to love them anyway and help them in any way you can. Find some way to support and help them, no matter how small and show them that you care and love them anyway. Keep the lines of communication open. If you don't, it could mean the end of a marriage, a relationship, or a family. What's it all worth to you?

Rhonda Byrne sends out inspirational e-mail messages periodically called *The Secret Daily Teachings.* Here's one that particularly resonated with me. "Trying to change someone is a waste of time. The very thought of changing someone is saying that they are not good enough as they are, and it is soaked with judgment and disapproval. That is not a thought of appreciation or love, and those thoughts will only bring separation between you and that person.

You must look for the good in people to have more of it appear. As you look only for the good things in a person, you will be amazed at what your new focus reveals." (Rhonda Byrne, personal communication)

Teach your children this very important lesson from *The Secret* so they will grow to appreciate diversity of all kinds. Stress kills. Make peace with people you've alienated or who've alienated you. Is it your wife, your husband, your brother, your sister, your mother, your father, a friend, a co-worker? Do it now before it's is too late. (Byrne 2006)

Attitude of Gratitude

I began by being thankful for having a second chance at living and for the alternative direction I chose. Then I confirmed my state of being every day by being grateful for all the opportunities, challenges, and gifts God was allowing me to experience and see, some for the first time in my life. Every challenge is a gift and an opportunity for growth in some area. Sometimes the transition, from here to there, is a bit scary.

Then I started to forgive everyone and everything that I felt was responsible for giving me an injustice of any kind, for these too have built-in benefits and opportunities. Ho'o pono pono to the rescue.

The release of these old paradigms created a sense of peace around me that felt great, yet unfamiliar. My attitude of gratitude was working. Peacefulness was setting in, so unusual, so welcome, and so beautiful. Even as I remember these things now, it brings me to a tearful, yet joyful place. I cry a lot of happy tears in this book, don't I? It's a really good place to be.

I never really felt anything from exchanging the sign of peace growing up as a Roman Catholic at church every Sunday. What did it really mean? After a lot of soul searching and reading about various spiritual teachings I did discover who I really was: a child of God and a child of the Universe. All, what I'll call non-traditional religious teachings, talked about unconditional love and forgiveness. None of them talked about sin, failure or fear. I began to realize my value, to know I had a place, no matter what it was. This was my God. No religion can extend that feeling. It has to come from inside, and until you feel it for yourself, you may not fully understand what I'm desperately trying to share with you here—no more guilt, no more feeling like a sinner, just real peace. It wasn't until I got breast cancer when I was fifty years of age and started to look at spirituality that I realized I wasn't going to purgatory or hell for dying with a so-called sin on my soul. I'm actually a bit embarrassed about that fact. Being a Roman Catholic really did a number on me.

When you love yourself unconditionally, you can easily love others unconditionally. What this means is to love yourself *more than your biggest* mistakes. To love someone else unconditionally is to love them *more than their biggest* mistakes. Thanks to Reverend Richard Rogers at Unity of Naples for that *ah ha* moment, which caused me to finally understand the true meaning of unconditional love. That's what makes the world go round, not just love, but unconditional love!

Speaking of Unity of Naples, what an amazing, uplifting service I attended recently. I continue to be blown away by the love I feel in this church community. There was a *tropical* theme that day to keep in line with Tropical Storm Isaac that was headed our way. A man played a steel drum beautifully, and the feature songs were "Day O" and, believe it or not, "Hot, Hot, Hot"! Go figure! Even though attendance was slim because of the impending storm, the roof was rocking! My ballroom dancing friend Debbie and I got up in the center aisle during "Hot, Hot, Hot" and did the Meringue! Can you believe it? What fun. This is the way *church* was meant to be, leaving people feeling uplifted and fulfilled! Hats off to Jodie, the music director, and Reverend Richard Rogers for continuing to make Unity of Naples a fabulous place to worship God, each other and a place of unconditional love!

I am 100 percent responsible for everything that comes into my moment, my day, my life, my world. What is going on inside me to manifest the things I do? Is it love? Is it fear? Is it hate? You harbor these feelings and emotions, then they become thoughts, then they become a belief system. When you let fear and hatred go, you will begin to truly live. Let the love grow stronger, let fear and hate melt away. Hey world, *I love you, I'm sorry, please forgive me, thank you!*

Patchouli

I have to share some lyrics to a beautiful song about forgiveness, written and composed by a favorite couple that I met when I moved to Naples. They call themselves Patchouli, with Julie Patchouli and Bruce Hecksel. From the City Pages review: "Nationally touring, award-winning songwriter Julie Patchouli and master guitarist Bruce Hecksel light up the air with sparkling acoustic sounds and their powerful contagious chemistry. Famous for that smiling voice that instantly turns a bad day into a good one, Patchouli's down-to-earth, hopeful songwriting is 'New American Folk,' blending elements of folk, pop, flamenco, and jazz with world-beat rhythms." (Patchouli "Patchouli's Band Biography" 2013)

Their music fills me up. Here are the lyrics to a very emotional song called "The Carrying" that Julie wrote about forgiveness. You can find it on their Woodlands CD and order it from their website. (Patchouli 2013)

"The Carrying"
Forgiveness, is such a strange thing
It makes the heart work, and the truth ring
It lets the day come, and the birds sing
A sweeter song, for the carrying
To the place where the broken go
To return to the ebb and the flow
Where the pieces again become whole
And holding, and we walk because if we run
We'll give ourselves away
We walk because if we run,
We'll give ourselves away.

If you ever feel called to extend forgiveness and need some encouragement, listen to this song. It will help to incite, motivate, and propel you to make amends with those who still need your love and need to know it.

Dr. Lorraine Day—Breast Cancer and Finding God

I mentioned Dr. Day back in Chapter 3 and she deserves another mention here. Dr. Day's complete healing occurred because of her spiritual connection to a positive belief system that involved forgiveness and love. All the alternative therapies she applied to recover from breast cancer, although extremely helpful, were not enough.

Her juicing, raw food and detoxing methods worked for a short while. She then got sick again, was bed ridden and couldn't even take nourishment by mouth any longer. Remembering that nutrition could be absorbed rectally through the colon, she began to use nutritional enemas. As she read her bible she realized there was a piece missing from a complete healing, love and forgiveness.

She realized that negative emotions create stress and stress can be very detrimental to your health. She let go of that stress by using forgiveness, appreciation, gratitude and practicing loving thoughts. Negative emotions that were in her heart kept her from recovering. The love and forgiveness that entered her heart after letting go of negative thoughts and feelings completed her wellness journey. How did she do it? She gave up bitterness, anger and resentment for pure love. Dr. Day is now seventy-four and looks fabulous.

Deepak Chopra

Deepak Chopra is a well-respected medical doctor and writer and he publishes extensively on spirituality and diverse topics in mind-body medicine. He's says: "Keep in mind that your cells are eavesdropping on what you say, so unless you want to have your father's bad back or anything else that "runs in the family," don't nurture that seed of intention in your awareness." (Chopra Center Newsletter "7 Secrets to Grow Younger, Live Longer" 2011)

Think of the consequences of that statement. Personally, I do believe every cell in my body is eavesdropping on my thoughts. That's why I choose to wake up each morning with a meditation and set my intentions. What intentions?—the tasks I expect to take on today and what I want the outcome to look like. I visualize everything as I want it to happen during my day. I take some time before each task and ask my spirit guides, my angels, my God, and the universe for guidance that the outcome will be favorable and in my best interest.

During my return to health, when I was preparing my food, doing a cleanse, reading, anything related to getting well, I always envisioned and *believed* I would completely overcome my cancer. I *believe* this process was significant in my ultimate return to health, if not *the* reason for it.

CHAPTER 10

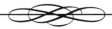

Enzymes

What Are Enzymes?

Enzymes are the elixir of longevity. They're not pure liquid, but they are pure gold in terms of the value they have to your life—not just your health, but your life. They are so precious that life anywhere in any form cannot live without them. Scientifically they are protein molecules manufactured by all plant and animal cells and catalysts that make chemical reactions go faster, but are not changed by the reaction. All cells require enzymes to survive and function.

Low Enzyme Content

Research has shown people who have a chronic disease or have low energy levels also have lower enzyme content in their blood, urine, and tissues. While there is clearly a direct relationship between disease states and a person's enzyme levels, only recently has the nature of that relationship been better understood. Researchers began to question whether a person's enzyme levels were low because they were sick, or whether they were sick because their enzymes levels were low.

The old thinking was *I am sick; therefore my enzyme levels are low.* The new thinking is *my enzyme levels are low, therefore I am sick.*

Enzymes are more important than the air you breathe, the water you drink, or the food you eat because without enzymes you wouldn't be able to breathe, swallow, drink, eat, or digest your food.

Many illnesses are the result of digestive problems, which create toxemia inside the body. Toxemia is the result of insufficient enzymes to properly digest and metabolize nutrients. If you aren't getting the nutrition from the food you eat, your body begins to break down and die a slow death from things that are otherwise directly under your control, namely, your diet.

Think about this for a minute. Have you ever been to your doctor with a sickness for anything simple like a cold and have the doctor say to you, "You need more enzymes"? I never have. Not even after I was diagnosed with breast cancer. If enzymes are so important to your health, and I believe they are, then why aren't doctors prescribing enzyme supplements, juicing and eat more raw foods? That's too easy, painless, and cost effective, right?

Enzymes Are Your Body's Workers

Enzymes are responsible for constructing, synthesizing, carrying, dispensing, delivering, and eliminating the many ingredients and chemicals the body uses in its daily business of living. Enzymes in raw food can be absorbed and used by our cells to replenish our stock of protein catalysts and help us digest our food. Enzymes are the catalysts for every metabolic reaction in our bodies. Without enzymes there can be no cell division, energy production, or brain activity. No brain activity without enzymes—can you imagine that?

Why do we consume foods that have little or no enzymes? We just don't know these essential scientific facts. Who in food manufacturing would tell you this? They want you to purchase their dead, over-processed, bottled, canned, and frozen foods. In order for food manufacturers to safely bottle and can foods, the foods must be heated to at least 212 degrees for fruits and 240 degrees for just about everything else in order to give these products shelf life of up to a year and longer. As a result, bottled and canned foods are lifeless, useless, and empty of nutrients because enzymes are destroyed at or around 118 degrees.

We have become communities fixated on convenient, extremely processed fast food, taking in way too much sugar and fat. Quite simply, this type of food demands excessive amounts of enzymes to digest, since the food itself does not contain enzymes. All the enzymes to digest this food are coming from our digestive and metabolic systems. As we continue our unhealthy eating habits, we deplete our enzyme stores, and then we age faster, get sick, and wonder why this has to happen to us. We are *processed food junkies.*

People in various communities are beginning to wake up, however, because many urban locations are finding ways to transform vacant city lots and rooftops into sustainable, organic, living vegetable and fruit gardens that can feed many people. This is happening all over the world, including urban city locations like Chicago, Milwaukee, New York City, and in Cuba. How cool is that!

Metabolic Enzymes

All organs and tissues are run by metabolic enzymes. Metabolic enzymes exist all over our body in all our organs, bones, and blood, and inside every cell. These enzymes are necessary in the growth of new cells and sustaining all tissue. Every organ has its own group of specialized enzymes trained to run and maintain that organ. When enzymes are healthy and plentiful, they perform well in doing the job they were designed to do.

Digestive Enzymes

Digestive enzymes are secreted by the salivary glands, stomach, pancreas, and the small intestine and help with breaking down proteins, carbohydrates, and fats. Digestive enzymes are also regarded as metabolic enzymes whose role is to digest food. One good thing about digestive enzymes is that they can be supplemented from an outside source if necessary.

Food Enzymes

Food enzymes, which are in raw fruits and vegetables, begin the process of digestion and are already naturally present within the food you eat, if you eat a raw food diet. *Cooking food at temperatures at or around 118 degrees destroys the enzymes.*

Digestive and food enzymes essentially serve the same function: to digest our food so it can be absorbed through the walls of our small intestine and into the bloodstream. From this perspective the only real difference between digestive and food enzymes is whether they originate from the raw food you eat or from inside your body.

Why Are Enzymes Important for Digestion?

Most raw foods contain enough natural food enzymes to digest that particular food. When you cook food, the enzymes are changed, inactivated, or destroyed and can no longer assist in digestion. When you eat cooked food your body becomes stressed and must create internally enough digestive enzymes to complete the digestive task. Your internal organs then have less time for rebuilding and replacing tired old cells that keep your immune system strong.

Your Body's Top Priority

Digesting food and assimilating the nutrients are your body's top priorities to make sure it has enough nutrients to keep it running. This takes a lot of energy and enzymes, especially if the body is required to meet the enzyme demand on its own.

It has been suggested that 70-80 percent of our body's energy is expended by the digestive process and because enzymatic action is required for our systems to function that we should take enzyme supplements.

Enzymes—Infinite Supply?

Until recently, many within the scientific community labored under the misconception that digestive enzymes in the body are constant and last forever, that they can be used and reused, and that they never get old and never wear out.

Researchers now know we lose digestive enzymes through sweat and body waste. As we age, organs responsible for digestive enzyme production become less efficient. Air and water pollution, overly processed foods, fast foods, genetically modified foods, and microwave cooking can result in free radical damage, which lowers the body's effectiveness in developing enzymes.

Enzyme Deficiency = Stressed Body

Your body works overtime to create the necessary enzymes to digest your food. This extra stress negatively impacts the immune system's ability to protect itself from and fight off disease. The body becomes so overtaxed it can't generate enough enzymes to properly digest your food. Undigested food particles then begin to pollute your body, and the chances of chronic disease increase. You get plenty of enzymes from a raw, live-food diet of fresh fruits and vegetables.

What is Raw, Living Food?

Uncooked, unprocessed, additive-free raw fruits and vegetables in their just-picked natural state are considered raw, living foods. This includes raw nuts, seeds, and sprouts.

118 Degrees—the Tipping Point

The thermal death point of living substances is around 118 degrees, which also blisters skin and prevents seed germination when seeds are exposed for a half hour or more. Enzymes do not have a chance to survive under any cooking method in which heat over 118 degrees is applied. This renders them useless for further breaking down food particles and nourishing our bodies.

Any cooking method—including slow or fast baking, boiling, stewing, frying, micro-waving, poaching, and barbecuing—destroys food enzymes. Frying and barbecuing also damage proteins and form new chemical compounds. These new chemical compounds could create new bacteria and disease, imposing yet more burdens upon metabolic enzymes. Bottom line:

COOKED FOOD equals **DEAD FOOD** equals **A DEAD BODY**

Solution

The solution, very simply, is to eat a predominantly organic, raw, plant-based diet. Eliminate processed, junk, and salty or sugary food and snacks! When you do have a cooked-food meal, add a good digestive enzyme supplement for better digestion and absorption.

An incredible resource to learn about enzymes is *Enzyme Nutrition, The Food Enzyme Concept* by Dr. Edward Howell. (Howell 1985)

Chapter 11

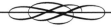

The Road to Health

Organic Versus Conventional Produce

It was a Sunday, and my favorite organic grocery store was closed. Literally everything in this store is organic, and you don't have to worry about whether you're looking at organic or conventionally grown produce in this market. It's all organic 100 percent of the time. There's even a sign above the produce department that says: "We are militantly organic so you can shop in peace." I was disappointed I didn't get groceries on Saturday. I was on my way home from the beach and was hot, thirsty, hungry and in need of some hydration and sustenance. (Food and Thought 2013)

I stopped at a farmer's market-type grocery store, which was on my way home, a place I don't normally shop. Wouldn't you know the first aisle in the produce department had all kinds of fresh fruit cut up for sampling, so organic or not, I caved in and sampled tangerines, cantaloupe, and watermelon, all very sweet and satisfying. Then I went about doing some vegetable shopping. I came across organic carrots, celery, and broccoli. Yippee! I needed a lot of carrots and celery, as I was beginning a detox the next day and was going to be juicing like crazy. So I then made my way to the onions and other vegetables, when I saw the produce manager.

I said, "Say, can I ask you a question"?

Of course he said yes. I asked why there wasn't more organic produce being sold at this store. He told me about the high price of produce and the clientele who shopped there and ultimately why they had to keep prices low. He then suggested I go to the store I mentioned above, where everything is organic.

I said, "Yes, I know that store very well, but it's closed on Sunday."

He knew that but at least wanted me to be aware of it in case I wasn't.

Then we got into a discussion about organic versus conventionally grown produce. He is a conventional-produce farmer and so is the rest of his family. He flat out told me the chemical pesticides, fertilizers, and fungicides they use on their crops are *POISON,* and all the conventional farmers know it.

"We use it anyway," he said.

I guess it's for the purpose of yielding larger crops that are more insect and mildew resistant. At whose expense? Yours and mine.

Where in the world has the moral aspect of farming gone? Why are we buying and supporting conventional farming when we know that poisons are being used to cultivate and grow our food supply. Follow the money!

I understand that when a farmer with integrity wants to switch his farming methods from conventional to USDA Certified Organic, there is a timely and expensive process to go through before the same land that was used for conventional farming can now be used for certified organic farming.

The Farming Systems Trial from 1981 to 2011 of organic versus conventional farming was completed by the Rodale Institute, which concluded the following: "The hallmark of a truly sustainable system is its ability to regenerate itself. When it comes to farming, the key to sustainable agriculture is healthy soil, since this is the foundation for present and future growth...After 30 years of side-by-side research in our Farming Systems Trial (FST)®, Rodale Institute has demonstrated that organic farming is better equipped to feed us now and well into the ever changing future."

Fast Facts

Organic yields match conventional yields.
Organic outperforms conventional in years of drought.
Organic farming systems build rather than deplete soil organic matter,
making it a more sustainable system.
Organic farming uses 45% less energy and is more efficient.
Conventional systems produce 40% more greenhouse gases.
Organic farming systems are more profitable than conventional.

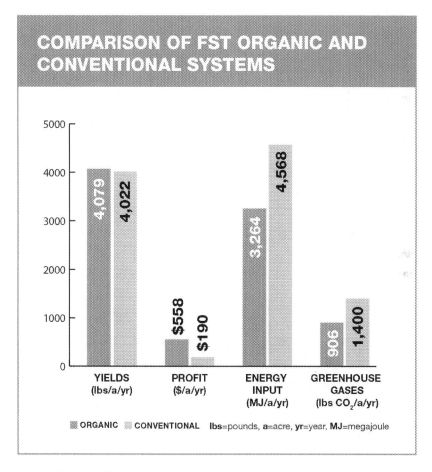

Copyright © Rodale Institute. Reprinted from the report "The Farming Systems Trial: Celebrating 30 years."

You can learn more about the Rodale Institute and review a complete copy of the study at the Rodale Institute website. (Rodale Institute "The Farming Systems Trial: Celebrating 30 years" 2013)

These statistics make it clear that there is no excuse for conventional farming to even exist any longer. This thirty-year study proves organic farming is better all around for the planet, for humanity, for future generations, and, more importantly, long-term sustainability than conventional farming.

I am often asked, "Is there that big a difference between organic and conventional produce?"

The answer is an absolute yes! Not just in the nutritional quality of the produce, but also in the flavor. You can tell the difference, especially after you've gone through a detox and your taste buds now recognize the true flavor of food and not the artificial food products you used to eat.

Everything that goes into growing organic produce is a creation of Mother Nature. Every cell in your body can benefit from it. Conventional produce contains chemicals, poisons, and toxins that your body just looks at and says, "What the heck do you want me to do with these? What are they?" So they sometimes are stored as garbage in your liver and other various organs and later turn into a disease if you have a weakened immune system.

Organic foods have 30 to 55 percent more vitamins and minerals in them than non-organic foods, and they're grown without chemical fertilizers and pesticides. I've heard some comments from folks complaining that organically grown produce is more expensive than their conventional counterparts. While that may be true in some cases, it depends on where you shop. You can shop at farmers' markets, belong to organic food co-operatives, and watch for sales on organic produce at your regular grocery store. Ultimately you can have a lower or equal produce cost with a higher nutritional value. Also, when you add in the cost of co-pays for doctor's office visits, co-pays for prescription drugs, gas and wear and tear on your car going to and from the doctor's office, the cost for organic produce becomes considerably lower. If you then add the value of the sick leave time you'll need from your employer to get to your doctor's appointments and the physical nature of just feeling lousy, organic produce is a bargain at any cost. Organic produce doesn't last as long in your refrigerator either. What does that tell you? Is the extra cost for organic produce worth it? Is your life worth it? You bet it is! As a once conventional farmer who turned to organic farming, Frank Oakes, owner of Food & Thought, posted a very revealing short video on his website about the differences between conventional and organic farming and the nutrient density of organically grown produce. Please take a look at it and know that organic produce is better for you in every way. (Food & Thought "Why Organic" 2013)

We came from the earth, we are a human form of vitamins, minerals, proteins and amino acids, all taking on the form of various bones, joints, skin, organs, and very complicated systems of liquid and solid food absorption, natural cleansing, blood purification, waste disposal, mental and motor connections, and communication. Our bodies depend on a steady supply of nutrient-dense food sources to keep these systems alive and in peak performance. When we feed our bodies with the chemical soup I see people put in their grocery carts, we deprive our bodies of the substances they so long for to keep healthy and vibrant. No wonder we are sick and diseased.

So what conclusion would you draw about the value of a predominantly raw, organic plant based diet and your health? Please don't tell me my story is anecdotal. That's what the doctors would want you to believe. The doctors can't say for sure what *caused* my *cure* because I wasn't part of any double-blind placebo-based study to prove it. But I know. I know the effects of a raw food diet and lifestyle change cured my cancer, or I wouldn't be in this fabulous vibrant state of health. Believe me, it was and is a complete and total cure.

There are thousands of people like me, some of whom have testimonials in the last chapter of this book, who were in the same boat. These people recovered from major diseases simply by changing their diet, their lifestyle, and their thoughts. *Change your diet, change your life!*

Anthony Gucciardi, co-founder of Natural Society.com, editor and investigative journalist talks about the contradictions discovered in a recent report put out by Stanford University claiming there is no difference between organic and conventionally grown produce. You'll be surprised to see who and what organizations were behind the report. (Maybe you won't be surprised.) You can hear what he has to say in the following video. (Gucciardi "Is There Really a Difference Between Organic and Conventional Food?" 2012)

Are We Fruitarians?

It's interesting that a much older male friend of mine used to be a fruitarian. He ate only fruit at each meal—breakfast, lunch, dinner, and snacks. He shared with me that when he practiced this fruit only diet he actually felt and looked better and was physically the strongest of any time in his life. So could some of us be fruitarians and not just vegans or vegetarians? Could some of us actually be meant to thrive on just fruit alone? Here is a look at some information that may offer yet another view into how a major change in your diet could create incredible wellness and vitality.

Dr. Douglas N. Graham, an author of many books, a lifetime athlete, an advisor to world class athletes, and a twenty-seven-year raw foodist, suggests that we are not meat eaters since we don't have sharp teeth to tear apart the flesh like some carnivorous domesticated and wild animals. He also suggests that we are not tubers, like animals that forage for their food underground, because we lack the sharp nails to dig through the sometimes hard dirt to get at potatoes, beets, and other produce that grows deep in and under the ground.

He does, however, suggest that because of the shape of our hands, our teeth, our long arms, and our two-legged stature we are easily designed to pick and eat fruit from just about any tree, bush, or plant that would grow above ground. Dr. Graham wrote a book called *The 80/10/10 Diet*, which focuses exclusively on mostly raw fruits and some vegetables. As you may know, some produce that we think of as vegetables, like tomatoes and cucumbers, are actually fruit.

Under Dr. Graham's diet plan you eat mega meals of fruit and vegetables.

For example, for breakfast you may consume two pounds of plums or four pounds of casaba melon. At lunch you would have two pounds of mango and eight ounces of butter lettuce with a squeeze of lime for some tang. Or, you might eat one pound of bananas, one pound of peaches, and eight ounces of blueberries. Dinner would be three large courses—a salad starter, a raw soup, and some other kind of big salad. None of his recipes include added fats, butters, or oils. Imagine that!

There's no meat in this diet plan, and there's a whole chapter of testimonials by people who've regained their health and athletes who've never felt better training and eating this kind of diet. (Graham 2006)

How to Eat Fruit and Drink Fruit Juices

Fresh fruit should be eaten on an empty stomach, either thirty minutes or more before a meal or several hours after. Fruit digests quickly and easily, as long as there are no other carbohydrates or proteins in your stomach to inhibit the process.

There is a lot of natural sugar in fruit, and when fruit is combined with other foods it begins to ferment and rot, causing gas, bloating, and other digestive disorders. The same is true for drinking any kind of fruit juice, whether fresh, canned or bottled. These juices should be consumed only on an empty stomach for the same reasons and to maximize nutrient absorption.

Drinking Liquids during Meals

Drinking cold or ice-cold anything, including water, before, during, or after meals is not advisable. Cold water solidifies the fats and oils in the meal you've just consumed, creating a sludge that slows down the digestion process. Sipping small amounts of room-temperature water or hot tea as needed to help you wash down your meal is really all that's necessary. Also, drinking large amounts of fluids before or during a meal dilutes the hydrochloric acid in your stomach and other digestive enzymes that are the key to breaking down your food into smaller particles in preparation for digestion and nutrient absorption.

Chew Your Food

The best way to consume a meal for optimum overall nutrient absorption is to chew each mouthful of food approximately thirty times so that it feels really smooth and mushy as you swallow. As you chew, enzymes are released from your saliva, which helps to initiate the digestion process even before your food actually reaches your stomach. When the food gets to your stomach, the hydrochloric acid and other digestive enzymes have a much easier job of further breaking it down into smaller particles for maximum nutrient absorption. You also have more frequent and easier bowel movements.

Drink Plenty of Pure, Fresh Water

Because our bodies are composed of around 70 percent water, everyone should drink at least half their body weight in ounces of water each day. Coffee, alcohol, and other liquids don't count. They just deplete your electrolytes. However herbal teas are good, especially green tea and other organic, non-caffeinated varieties that are loaded with antioxidants.

When you're used to drinking pure water, you'll never be able to go back to drinking tap water again. I live in southwest Florida and attended a dance party that was held outside in the middle of the summer. The temperature was 90 degrees with relatively high humidity. There were about seventy people at this dance, and everyone was sweaty, hot, and sticky, having a ball dancing up a storm anyway. I had already run out of the one container of water I brought with me and was dying of thirst. I went to the nearest water fountain and didn't even think of what I might experience. I took one long gulp and then said, "Oh, My God, this is terrible."

The chlorine smell and taste was so strong I couldn't drink any more, even though I desperately needed more hydration.

When you get used to drinking pure water from whatever system you invest in, you won't be able to tolerate anything else. Your body will like it, too!

Toxic Water Solutions

Purchase a whole-house, water-purification and alkalizing system for your home. Use a brand of bottled, reverse-osmosis water or some other brand of deep-well, bottled water, like those that come from Fiji, to take with you when you travel, or bring your own from your home system.

If you can't afford to get a whole-house, water-purification system, get shower filters to take out chlorine and other toxic chemicals and dechlorinating bath salts for your bath water. Or you can fill up your bath with the water from the shower, if you have a combined bathtub shower area.

You can also purchase many of these products from the big-box, home-improvement centers, health-food stores, or online.

Toxic Air Solutions

While we can't do much about the air we breathe outside of our homes or in our cars, we can take some steps to clean the air we breathe in our homes, where we take at least 33 percent of our breaths.

Get a whole-house, air-filtration system for your furnace and air conditioner with an electronic cleaning device. If you can get it, add on to this system a device that generates negative ions that nature uses to clear the air of dust and other particles and also produces activated oxygen to remove odors without the use of fragrances. There are smaller devices available commercially if a whole-house system is cost prohibitive.

Get a humidifier for the same system, if you live in a cold and dry climate and you're running the heat or your wood stove all winter long. Prolonged heating can dry out your furniture, your belongings, and your body. Purchasing a humidifier will help keep both you and your household furnishings hydrated, especially in the winter, depending on geographic location.

You can also purchase some Himalayan Salt Lamps. These also produce negative ions to counteract harmful positive ions that are created from the use of electronic devices of all kinds.

Animal Protein—A Final Note

Dr. Campbell's book, *The China Study*, was all the proof I needed to eliminate all red meat and most dairy products from my diet. I occasionally enjoy a piece of wild salmon or free-range chicken. The free-range chicken is grown with feed that's been processed without the use of chemical fertilizers, herbicides, or pesticides. If you choose to eat red meat after reading this book, please be sure to buy red meat that has been 100 percent grass-fed and allowed to roam freely in the pastures. If you elect to eat fish, be sure it's wild. If you eat chicken or white-meat options, again, be sure the animals are allowed to roam freely, treated humanely and are fed organic feed. And make it only 5 percent or less of your diet. (Campbell and Campbell 2005)

Here's an interesting short story. I went home to Bennington, Vermont, one year for Thanksgiving. My sister and brother-in-law have the most beautiful chocolate Lab with the softest ears, the deepest brown eyes, and the absolute most adorable smile and face. Yes, animals smile. He also has the most agreeable and docile of personalities you could ever imagine.

Patti didn't purchase an organic turkey that year, so she wasn't planning to use the turkey's insides (heart, liver, and gizzards) in the gravy. Instead she offered the liver to Red, the chocolate lab. We were dumfounded as Red was excited, jumping up and down and wagging his tail from side to side, thinking he was going to get a real treat. Patti put the plate down in front of him. He smelled the liver, lifted his head, looked at us, turned his nose up in the air and walked away, leaving the liver completely untouched. It was almost like he was saying, "Hey, this stuff is poison, and there's no way I'm going to eat it. I don't care how good it looks."

My brother-in-law, nephew, and a few other relatives are all avid deer hunters, and my sister had a deer liver in the freezer, so, just as an experiment, she took it out and defrosted it. A few hours later after the liver thawed and reached room temperature, she once again tried to feed Red a liver, but this time from a wild deer, not a turkey.

Red *wolfed* that liver down so quickly it was amazing. This dog does not suffer from hunger, ever, so it's not like he was full and wasn't hungry when offered the non-organic, toxic, turkey liver and starving when offered the wild deer liver.

Red knew. He could smell the difference between something that was healthy and something that was toxic. Red was sniffing all the chemical fertilizers, pesticides, and fungicides that were used in the food supply and given to the turkey while it was being farmed. He couldn't smell any of those things in the deer liver because there weren't any there to detect.

If you do choose to eat animal protein, please be sure it's grass-fed, free range, and in the case of fish or other proteins from the oceans, wild caught or in some way organically grown and cared for. And as Dr. Campbell suggests, keep it to a 5 percent maximum of your diet.

The Problem with Dairy

All milk today processed for human consumption is pasteurized or ultra-pasteurized and is heated to temperatures of 161 degrees for regular pasteurization and for a shorter time to 275 degrees for the ultra-pasteurized products. This process destroys any bacteria contained in the milk. The problem is that it also destroys any natural enzymes and most, if not all, of any nutrient value it may contain.

Many people are allergic to milk or have trouble digesting it because as humans we lack the digestive enzymes necessary to break down and utilize cow's milk once ingested. Baby cows were meant to drink cow's milk; human babies were meant to drink human milk from their mother's breast. Humans are the only animals on earth to consume the milk of another animal. Isn't there a point here?

In repeated laboratory experiments calves fed *pasteurized* milk for sixty days die. Repeat: in repeated laboratory experiments calves fed *pasteurized* milk for sixty days die. Pasteurized milk is dead milk. It has no nutritional value; therefore, animals that drink it will die.

Milk turns to an acid once in our stomachs. Your body needs to stay alkaline to stay alive. When you drink or eat anything that's acid, your body stands at attention and says, "Ok, alkalize or die." So the body, desperately wanting to live, (it's very intelligent) looks to become alkaline again. Alkalizing minerals are calcium, phosphorous, and magnesium. Where are these alkalizing minerals located in your body? They come from your bones, teeth, and muscles. After your body retrieves the alkalizing minerals from your bones, teeth, and muscles, your bones, teeth and muscles begin to weaken because they've been robbed of nutrients that keep them strong.

What happens to the excess calcium and magnesium running through your bloodstream? It gets deposited in areas of your body where it isn't supposed to be, like the walls inside your arteries and into the joints of your fingers, hips, toes and knees, setting the stage heart disease and arthritis.

So the actual process of consuming calcium in the form of dairy products counteracts the very reason we drink or eat them to begin with. Any alternative health-care professional will tell you this. Drinking pasteurized cow's milk begins the process of arteriosclerosis, which is hardening of the arteries; arthritis; and unnecessary excessive buildup of calcium deposits in places where they don't belong.

Cow's milk contains an enzyme called xanthine oxidase, which, after the homogenization process, can be absorbed into our bloodstream through the intestinal walls. These xanthine oxidase enzymes are sticky and can build up on the wall of your arteries and could be deposited in other places like in between joints, where it doesn't belong. Human breast milk does not contain this enzyme, so mothers breast feeding their babies don't need to worry about human-breast milk. It has just the right ingredients for that little baby. Cow's milk is for calves, not humans.

You can get all the calcium and protein you need from dark-green, leafy vegetables. Cows eat grass and drink water. Horses eat grass and drink water. Elephants eat grass and drink water. All these animals eat grass and drink water to grow strong bones and muscle tissue. They don't eat meat or dairy products from other animals. You can eat grass and other leafy greens and drink water, too, and stay younger and healthier than you could ever imagine.

Drinking cow's milk or consuming other dairy products is a recipe for sickness, especially in the heart disease area, whether you are six weeks or sixty years old. Tell me once again, why are we drinking pasteurized cow's milk and eating cheese? (Mercola.com "Does Milk Really Look Good On You" 2013)

Read the Labels

You know that old saying, "If you can't pronounce what's in it, then you probably don't want it in or on you"? Whoever came up with that saying deserves a Nobel Prize. You can reduce your exposure to some major toxins if you just read the label and make smarter choices. We always have another choice, even if it's to eliminate the purchase altogether.

You might say, "But this food is being sold in the USA, and all of the ingredients must have been approved by the Food and Drug Administration, so they must be safe and harmless to consume, right?"

Well, you can do the research yourself, but I'm suggesting that not all is well with the FDA. Based on books I've read, stories I've listened to, and documentaries I've watched, we have a huge body of government employees who allow food additives to be approved that are not safe, no matter what the quantity is in the product being produced.

Here are the ingredients in a popular brand of buttery spread compared to an organic butter.

Popular Buttery Spread: Vegetable oil blend (soybean, palm, and palm kernel oil), water, whey (milk), salt, mono and diglycerides, soy lecithin, (potassium sorbate, calcium disodium EDTA) used to protect quality, citric acid, vitamin A palmitate, beta carotene (color), natural and artificial flavor, cholecalciforal (vitamin D3). Contains milk (whey) and soy, gluten-free. Total ingredients = *thirteen*

Organic Butter: Pasteurized organic sweet cream (mild), salt without flowing agents.

Total ingredients = *two*

You choose: two or thirteen? If they need to add *color* to make it look like butter and some chemical to protect the *quality* and they add natural and artificial flavors, just what is this stuff made from? More importantly, what are all those unidentifiable food ingredients doing to your insides? What would the quality be like if they didn't put the ingredient in there to *protect quality*? I guess they try to make you believe there was quality there to begin with. Hmmm?

Yes, I see the ingredient list, and you may think, *Gee, it doesn't seem that bad to me.* But remember, this is just one item in your refrigerator. When you repeat this process with every meal and snack, where do you think these toxins go? Your body doesn't recognize these ingredients, so it can't assimilate them into anything usable for regenerating and repairing cells to get and keep you healthy. So they frequently end up in your liver, your inside filter, and get stuck there among other places.

Let's not forget the packaging and the marketing. The tub of buttery spread looks so appealing with a lovely barn set in a sunny field promoting a good source of this vitamin and that vitamin. Makes you stop, look, and think, *Maybe this is good for me. It says so on the label. At least there are no hydrogenated oils in many of the margarine products being manufactured and sold today.*

Do you know where margarine came from? Take a look at the explanation on the Wikipedia website of how margarine is *manufactured*— yes, manufactured. You won't touch or buy it again. The description includes the following: "Commonly, the natural oils are hydrogenated by passing hydrogen through the oil in the presence of a nickel catalyst, under controlled conditions." Thank you, I've heard enough, not for me. (Wikipedia "Margarine" 2013)

This is interesting. There was an experiment a friend of mine did with a small bowl of butter and one of margarine. He put them both outside in the yard to see what the birds and animals would do. Well, it was really no surprise, because the birds and animals left the bowl of margarine untouched, and it didn't even turn brown or grow mold or anything else on it. He lives in Florida; it gets hot there. The bowl of butter had all kinds of birds and bugs dipping into it. No surprise, the butter disappeared.

Why didn't the birds, bugs, and other critters eat the margarine? I believe it was the chemical additives and the artificial ingredients. Just like Red, the chocolate Lab, animals and insects have keen instincts. They know what's healthy and what isn't, and they won't consume anything that's bad for them. It's that simple. I should ask my sister to do a test like that with Red! I bet he wouldn't touch the margarine but he would *wolf* down the butter.

Too bad most of us humans don't have that same keen instinct and intuition as animals do. We'd be a lot healthier.

Toxic Lifestyle Solutions

Throw out your microwave, stop smoking or drinking excessively, and give up your drugs and medications as much as possible. Get some exercise so you can sleep better; give up your stressful lifestyle and reclaim your health.

Microwaves change the molecular structure of every living thing cooked in one. They kill the nature of the food you're consuming, and one thing you don't need is to eat more dead food that your body can't use. Check out what Dr. Mercola has to say about the perils of using a microwave oven and why the Russians banned them. (Mercola.com "Why did the Russians Ban an Appliance Found in 90% of American Homes?" 2013)

Accept Who You Are

Do you really need breast implants or plastic surgery to feel good about yourself? It's only when we have low self-esteem to begin with, that we look outside of ourselves for acceptance. Once you start loving who you are—every single, delicious morsel of who you are—you will begin to realize that you don't need to live for anyone else except you.

Three of my girlfriends came to visit recently, and we're all big supporters of a raw food lifestyle, some more than others. But one thing we talked about was the pressure that's put on us, particularly women, by various manufacturers, big business, and companies with a product or service to sell primarily to women. They do this by getting us to believe we need their product to live, look good, and be healthy. We get sucked into their advertising for whiter teeth, makeup products, and getting rid of unsightly veins on our legs. And why not? Wow! Who wouldn't want to look like these women? The models they use— with their long, thin beautiful bodies, slinky hair, painted nails and toes, and shapely legs—cause us to believe using their products will transform us. Do these products really work that way? Of course not.

You have a beautiful, God-given body and composition that are uniquely yours. It's what's going on inside of you that is causing you to feel like you need to succumb to these products when maybe all you need to do is rework what you do with your food intake, your work, your family, and your friends.

You are beautiful just the way you are! Start feeding your way to better health by what you put inside your body, and you will radiate on the outside. Raw food can transform you on the inside and out

I was out dancing the other night when I met a woman, in her eighties, who told me I had beautiful skin. I was shocked. Not that I don't think I do have great skin, just that I'm au naturel. I wear no makeup, except sometimes a natural hemp lipstick. And you won't believe what I use besides a raw food diet to help my skin look and feel so good. It is flax, olive, avocado, and coconut oils. Yup—plain old certified organic, cold-pressed, unrefined, gluten-free, and non-GMO flax, olive, avocado, and coconut oils. I put a little on a warm, wet face cloth and apply gently to my face and neck, and my skin instantly absorbs the nutrients like a sponge. You must keep flax oil in the refrigerator because it can spoil quickly. How's that for a beauty treatment? I love it! It's inexpensive; I can use it on my skin, or in my salad dressings and smoothies, or just to take a tablespoon of flax oil once a day straight out of the bottle. Flax oil has a high concentration of omega 3's, and that's one thing we need to heal diseased cells in our body and keep the good ones we have working at peak efficiency. Rub some avocado oil on your feet and then cover them with a pair of cotton socks over night and you'll wake up with the softest feet ever.

Sorry, ladies, I want to look like me. The slightly wider-hipped, beat up shins, double wide-footed, five-foot-six-inch tall woman I am, not like someone else's version of what I should look like. All of those things I just recently learned to love about myself caused a whole new world to open for me. Learn to love, honor, and respect who you are inside and out, and the rest of your life will just fall into place. (I will admit, though, I do color my hair. I just can't get by the whole salt and pepper thing yet. I'm still a work in progress, too!)

Let's stop some of these bad habits and buying products that may be very harmful to our bodies. We can all *but* ourselves to death and *excuse* our way into believing that someone else has control over our decisions and destiny to make healthy changes in our lives, right? I used to say that too. *But* we are totally in charge and responsible. Don't give yourself away to advertising assaults and marking madness.

Whenever I go away I sometimes excuse myself from my usual lovely diet and lifestyle and say, "Oh, I'm on vacation, I can have a treat," and "I'll get back on track when I get home." Sound familiar? The truth is a treat now and then isn't going to hurt or harm you unless it becomes a trigger and puts you completely back into your old eating and lifestyle habits. Only you can decide how often and how much you stray from your new sustainable way of living.

We all have stress in our lives, and how many people do you know who've given up alcohol or tobacco, for example (no small task to say the least), been clean for a while, and suddenly they fall back into it? And the excuse they give is that they were undergoing a lot of stress at a certain time for this reason or that reason. It was the holidays, or I'm having a bad time at work, and so that makes it OK to eat a lot of junk food or the wrong food and start smoking or drinking again. I'm not judging anyone here; I'm trying to make a point that no one can overdose on a toxic load of physical, mental, and emotional stressors and avoid a sickened, malfunctioning immune system.

The goal here is to make you so in love with the new you and your new lifestyle you've just created that you won't ever care to fall back into old destructive habits again.

"STOP IT!"

You may remember Bob Newhart, the dry-humored and very funny comedian who played the role of a psychologist on his television shows. Well, he has a six-minute YouTube video that is hysterical. (OK, so I have a bizarre sense of humor.) But this woman comes to him with some fear-based problems, the largest of which is the fear of being buried alive in a box. In addition to that problem, she's also bulimic and has male relationship issues. She's quite surprised that the only solution he offers is for her to STOP IT! She attempts to go into a barrage of excuses about all the time she's been thinking about being buried alive in a box, how her bulimia problems started, and the fear that wells up in her every time she thinks about it. He just looks at her again and says, STOP IT! She persists and is very upset about the way her therapy session is going, so he tries to console her by saying he's going to give her ten words of advice and she should write them down. I quote him. He says: "Stop it or I'll bury you alive in a box!" (Newhart 2010)

So, while this may be an oversimplified version of trying to *stop* and overcome some really unhealthy lifestyle eating, drinking, work, and emotional habits, it's also very true. When you think about this, the decision is really that simple. The question is, are you ready for it? If and when you get to the point where you're sick to death of being sick to death and tired of continuously relying on doctors and their medications, you may well decide to stop it. Another approach will be like a breath of fresh air, and you will welcome it. Stop what you're doing and begin to look at and apply a different method of solving your health challenges and your fears.

CHAPTER 12

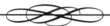

Belief

I N HIS BOOK *THE SPONTANEOUS Healing of Belief, Shattering the Paradigm of False Limits* Gregg Braden says: "Yes, we are occasionally victims of circumstance. And yes, we are sometimes the powerful creators of those same circumstances. Which of these roles we experience is determined by choices that we make in our lives, *choices based upon our beliefs.* Through the godlike power of human belief, we are given the equally divine ability to bring *what* we believe to life in the matrix of energy that bathes and surrounds us." (Braden 2008, xvii)

Belief

Thoughts are things we think.

What we think turns into a belief.

A belief creates a feeling.

A feeling produces a vibration.

Vibrations extend from us to those around us, our world, and the universe.

Like ripples in a pond and sound waves traveling throughout the universe, these vibrations represent your desires and your intentions.

Vibrations create the life we experience. Are yours going to be positive or negative?

Every positive and negative thought, word, deed, motion, and emotion is a vibration and goes out to every cell in your body and into the universe. These thoughts, words, deeds, motions, and emotions are creative energies. Do you want to create health and wellness? Or do you want to create disease and sickness? Whatever you think, believe, and feel, you create.

I'm going to get cancer, heart disease, diabetes, arthritis, etc. because it runs in my family. Aunt Jane died from lung cancer. Uncle Jim had triple bypass surgery and died anyway. Aunt Rachel is severely crippled with arthritis and osteoporosis, and my father had diabetes. I must be doomed, because *it all runs in my family.* You may as well sign a death sentence right now and get it over with.

> I am going to get cancer. I am going to get heart disease.

> I am healthy. I am well. I am vibrant. My body is performing perfectly.

Feel the difference? Either way, you are making a declaration about your state of health. You are making an emphatic and explicit proclamation of what you desire. All your thought vibrations go out to the universe and deliver back to you exactly what you believe you will get. Do you want vibrant health or debilitating disease? This is your choice, your choice and no one else's! You are the powerful creator of who you choose to be. *Your* thoughts, beliefs, and feelings, create your reality, not your family history.

You will create—repeat, you will create—whatever it is you are feeling based upon the vibrations you are expressing and sending out to the universe.

I cured myself from breast cancer. I am a powerful being of God; I know it, and I have proof. I'm living the proof every day. Did I need any double-blind placebo-based laboratory experiments to make me believe what I did was right for me or that the direction and the choices I made were working? No, and I still don't.

There is not much to learn about applying the techniques used to recover from any health condition. Visualize your body well and believe it already is. While this can be simply put, it may be difficult to understand, depending on where you are with your own belief systems. It also depends on your state of mind when you get a cancer diagnosis or other life-threatening disease that may throw you into a state of emotional trauma. Thoughts immediately turn to possibly dying, leaving family behind, and making out your will, health-care proxy and other legal documents you've put off for so long. Suddenly you have this incredible drive to make and act on the proverbial *bucket list* of things you always wanted to but didn't have the time, money, or the inclination. Now you have a reason because you may not be here tomorrow. How our perspective on life can change in an instant.

Life can be as eternal as you wish it to be. You just have to want it, focus on it, and *believe* you can have it, and you will.

Many spiritual authors talk of changing your thoughts, changing your life. It's true. A friend of mine recently gave me a framed piece of artwork which says: "The secret to having it all, is believing that you already do." Creating the image of it, seeing it materialize in your mind even before it does, is incredibly powerful.

We've been so brainwashed by the media from all walks of life, especially fear-based religions, into thinking we are guilty victims and that we must succumb to someone else's prescription for healing that we don't even know what to believe anymore. Look inside yourself for the answers, they are there.

In my own spiritual journey over the last seven-plus years I've been introduced to many spiritual teachings. As I studied each one, each one brought a new level of understanding and belief about who I am and why I'm here. The specifics of my particular journey are unimportant, but what is important is what I learned about the ultimate healing I received and why I continue to experience the highest level of health imaginable at this point in my life.

As I've mentioned, just a few times before, I don't take any prescription medications and no over-the-counter medications for anything. But, all that said, I've come to realize through the patterns expressed in almost every form of spirituality that there was one underlying significant commonality that always stood out. It was in the *believing* that a *healing* could take place that it can.

Why is it that some people can cure themselves of cancer using a macrobiotic diet, pureed asparagus, alkaline water, organic raw foods, and cottage cheese combined with flax seed oil or by watching comedy shows and movies and laughing themselves well, and other people who may employ those same cures are not cured?

In my opinion the underlying common denominator is *belief.* Each person who shared a testimonial of recovery using any of the methods listed above believed the program they were using was going to heal and cure them. Their state of mind turned from being a victim to taking full charge of what they were doing for themselves. They stopped being a victim. They gave up their fear-based life and became the powerful beings they knew in their hearts that they were. If we are made in the image and likeness of God, and we have God-like powers in us—why not use these powers to heal ourselves?

What each person had in common is that they took responsibility for their own lives, stopped playing the blame game, and got well. They took their God-like power back (from where ever it was) and applied it. They made the decision on which course of treatment to use and then *believed* it would work and it did.

The emotion and feeling of their new-found desire to believe these treatments would work caused them to become extraordinarily powerful. Their new-found freedom and independence from corporate and religious authorities created within them the desire to live. I suggest to you that whatever you decide to do under these circumstances cannot fail.

Healing of a Tooth

Florida farmers produce more than just citrus fruit. Our almost year-round sunshine allows us to grow some other great crops as well. In the summer of 2010 my friend Denise asked me to go blackberry picking with her and some other folks. I've mentioned not eating just one before, however, this time nature provides my attraction and affection for berries, all kinds, but particularly blackberries.

When you pick your own blackberries, or any kind of berries for that matter, I alternately eat one, save one. I ate at least as many blackberries as I had in my bucket before I was finished picking. These thornless blackberry bushes are organically grown and four-feet-high. That made for very easy picking. If that wasn't enough, the farm owners in their marketing foresight saw fit to provide each picker with a short elastic bungee-type cord with hooks on each end to wrap around your waist. Each hook would attach to one side of a one-gallon bucket handle that hangs in front of you so you have *both* hands free for picking. So guess what happened. Not one in the bucket, one in the mouth, but two in the bucket, two in the mouth.

Because my mother picked all kinds of berries, it seemed we were picking berries all summer long. My favorites were the sweet, large, juicy blackberries that grew on the Woodford Lake dirt roads on our way into our camp and down to the beach. The organic blackberries I picked with my friend were better than any I had ever eaten.

I ate enough blackberries that day for me to eliminate any further meals, but then there was always tomorrow! When tomorrow came I proceeded to dip my hand into the bucket and began a second fabulous feast all over again.

That's when it happened. I was chewing my blackberries when I felt a sharp pain in one of my upper left molars. As you may know, blackberries have seeds that only a car crusher could break open, and why I was trying to do this with my own teeth, God only knows. I think I was trying to enjoy every flavor morsel possible.

Sometime in the next few days I started to experience some discomfort in one of my upper left molars, so much so that I had to call a dentist. I went to a dentist in Ocala, and he took an X-ray but didn't see any crack or obvious tooth impairment. I knew something was wrong because when I pushed in toward my tongue with my finger there was sharp pain. Pushing outward toward my cheek, no pain. Hmmm? What was that all about? The dentist wasn't sure, either. He suspected a minor crack that wasn't even visible with an X-ray, so he decided to do a little drilling anyway and see if something became more apparent as he drilled. He found a *soft* patch under a filling and proceeded to take that out and filled it back up, hoping that would do the trick.

The next day I was in awful pain, called him, and went back. He still couldn't find anything really wrong with the tooth, so he drilled a little more beyond the last time and refilled it again. Next day, less pain but something was still there. I kept poking at it off and on. You know by now how I like to *poke* at things. Why do I do that?

I decided to go visit the biological dentist who had removed the second half of my amalgam fillings. This trip took me to Daytona Beach, Florida which was about a two hour drive from The Villages, Florida, where I used to live, but he was very good and I trusted him.

He found the same thing, nothing. He did give me some additional interesting information. He said he had a patient in the recent past that had a very small, almost undetectable minor crack in the root of one of his molars. He advised the patient of his options. One was to have the tooth pulled and a bridge put in to replace the missing tooth which would involve crowning each tooth on either side of the pulled tooth. The other was to wait it out and see if the life systems in and around the cracked tooth could rebuild the dentin inside the root and ultimately repair and heal itself.

Well the tooth did repair itself, and voila! The man was saved from having a tooth extracted and from spending all the time and money associated with having bridge work done. Isn't this a remarkable story? A tooth with a minor crack can actually repair itself with time and gentle caring.

My Daytona dentist also recommended that I have a crown put on that same tooth to keep it together, if and after it healed.

Again, I thought, *If someone else did it, I can do it just as well.* That's what I decided to do. I was going to wait it out and give the left side of my mouth plenty of rest from any chewing for six months to see what would happen. Except for very warm cooked foods and soups, that's exactly what I did. Now I'm a raw foodist, so just how much warm cooked food did I consume? Not much.

One month after another I would introduce denser foods to see how the tooth would react. After a while I discovered I was able to eat softer raw vegetables like zucchini and yellow squash, raw tomatoes, and some softer nuts like cashews and walnuts. Carrots would be the big test. When I could chew a raw carrot on that side of my mouth with little or no discomfort, I knew it was time for the next step.

I knew enough about the power of belief back then to activate and apply every aspect of it and visualization so I could to heal this tooth. I was sending out positive feelings, emotions and vibrations and each week my tooth got better and better. I believed I could and would heal it with a passion and the deepest emotion. I could cure breast cancer; a cracked tooth was a piece of cake!

During my meditation I would visualize chewing on that side of my mouth just the same as the other side, as though everything was quite normal, and then being in the dentist's chair undergoing the next phase of the repair. Well, that day finally came, and I'm happy to say I'm the proud owner of a healed upper left molar with a crown to keep it together.

Now here's the kicker, what really drove me. I was scared to death of having a tooth pulled. Don't ask me why, I just was. I didn't like the idea of somebody sticking a big old pair of stainless steel pliers in my mouth with their foot on the chair as they yanked out my tooth. That was a vision a friend of mine shared when he had a tooth pulled once. I guess it was a terrible experience, and the dentist did, in fact, put his foot on the chair while pulling the tooth.

The motivating factor was fear, but I turned that around to be a positive aspect in this example, and it worked for me. This was similar to thinking about using chemotherapy, radiation, and surgery to treat breast cancer. There was a lot of fear there too and that fear drove me to use alternatives to cure my cancer. I can't tell you how grateful I am to comfortably chew raw carrots, raw almonds, and Brazil nuts on that side of my mouth. Thanks to my ability to believe in the wholeness of who I am and what I accomplished with my breast cancer and now with my tooth, I no longer need convincing of the power we all possess if we just choose to use it.

Jet Lag

I was making plans to go to Palm Springs, California, where I was going to experience several spiritual tours of the desert with Frederic Delarue, the French author and music composer I previously mentioned. Once on his website click on the link for "Private Spiritual Tours of the Dessert." (Frederic Delarue 2012)

It takes the average person one full day to recover from each hour of time-zone change the body goes through. I'm the average person, or at least I thought I was. I've done a lot of international traveling and usually felt exhausted and worn out for several days before feeling normal again no matter which direction I was traveling. Time-zone changes have always been the most difficult part of long distance travel for me, especially when it involved several time zone changes at one time.

I was in Florida, and Frederic Delarue and the tours were in California, a three-hour time zone change away. I also had three take offs and landings starting in Fort Lauderdale at 1:00 p.m., changing planes in Austin, Texas and a final stopover in Oakland took me into the Ontario, California airport at 9:30 p.m. I was on East Coast time and my body thought it was 12:30 a.m., the next day. Palm Springs was about an hour drive south of Ontario.

I picked up my suitcase from the baggage claim area, picked up a rental car, drove to the hotel, and somehow was supposed to feel bright-eyed and bushy-tailed for noon the next day. A three-hour time zone change meant a three day recovery time period for me to feel good again under normal circumstances. I didn't have that much time. I was going to be in Palm Springs for just four full days, and Frederic's desert tours were scheduled for the first two days after my arrival. I wasn't keen on missing any part of the tours because I wasn't mentally alert enough to stay focused. Jet lag always made me feel foggy and light headed, and I would usually need a lot of rest before my body adjusted.

In addition to the jet lag problem, and what for me makes this testimonial to belief so powerful, are the other problems I had before I could get to sleep that night. After renting the only car left in the rental lot, a Volkswagen Beetle, and driving to Palm Springs at 11:00 p.m. over route I-10 and other unfamiliar roads, I arrived around midnight and checked into my hotel room.

A terrible chemical like odor was obvious. I called the front desk, and the only other room they had available was on the other side of the hotel. I decided I would try to tough it out. I woke up at 3:00 a.m. and couldn't tolerate the smell any longer. I called the front desk and suggested I take that other room, but first I wanted to smell it. If this odor was present in all the rooms, I was going to check out and go somewhere else. I inspected the other room, and thank God there was no chemical smell, so I moved there in the middle of the night. A male security guard came to help me relocate my things. Feeling like a vagabond in my PJ's without a bathrobe, toiletries in tow, I moved and settled into my second room in this hotel in less than four hours.

I set the alarm on my phone to 10:00 a.m. That would give me enough time to shower, have breakfast, and be ready at noon for my first tour with Frederic. I was so looking forward to this. Sleep finally came around 4:00 a.m.

I woke up to the sound of my phone, but it wasn't the alarm. It was my friend, Heidi, calling to say hello, but she didn't know I had plans to be in California so she was unaware of the three-hour time zone difference in our locations. After we talked a few minutes and said our good byes, I was awake but not coherent. No surprise there.

I thought if I was going to make anything of this day, I needed to get my act together and believe my way into feeling not just good but *great* and totally in synch with the new time zone. I didn't want to miss any part of this tour for any reason. This visit was already a rescheduled event from another time when I had made plans and had to cancel them.

I laid in bed and decided to meditate and visualize my body in an incredible state of awareness, alertness, total consciousness—wide awake, refreshed, feeling light, and completely in touch and in agreement with the Pacific Time Zone.

It happened! I think I even surprised myself. When I was finished meditating, about a half hour later, I got out of bed and felt fabulous. I took a shower, went to breakfast at the hotel, met Frederic in the lobby, and had just an absolutely glorious day. I didn't get back to my hotel until around 9:30 p.m. and was still feeling wonderful. I never did suffer any further effects of jet lag the rest of my time in Palm Springs.

You may not be able to completely understand just how profound this was for me unless you've experienced a similar situation. However, this my friends, is the power of *belief.*

Compelling Story of Feeling-Based Prayer—Belief

You may have seen the YouTube video in which Gregg Braden discusses the incredible power of belief as it pertained to a three-minute healing of a woman who was diagnosed with an inoperable, three-inch, bladder tumor. It's amazing how the combined power of energy and belief affected this healing. (Braden 2010)

As a last resort this woman went to a medicineless hospital in Beijing. The practitioners there taught her positive belief systems, breathing techniques, moderate exercise applications, and nourishing and healing ways to sustain her body.

In the video she is lying on a hospital bed, fully awake and conscious, and she believes the process about to take place will heal her. In an ultrasound split screen, you see on one side a still picture of the tumor as it was before the treatment she is about to receive. On the other side of the screen you see the real time image of the bladder tumor as an ultrasound technician moves the ultrasound wand over the tumor area.

There were three energy practitioners present who were trained in using their energy, the patient's energy, and a positive-belief system. They were able to utilize all that positive energy and feeling in conjunction with the woman's belief in order to actually eliminate her tumor, in just three minutes, without anesthesia or surgery. As the practitioners chanted, "already healed, already done," the woman believed that she was, in fact, already healed. All the positive energy being focused on her caused the tumor to melt away. You can watch the tumor actually melt away right before your eyes on this video.

Chapter Summary

How much more proof do we need that indeed our belief system affects our health as well as every other area of our lives? If you want to supercharge your life with positive thoughts and feelings that will create, construct and support a vibrant life, all you have to do is believe in those positive aspects and that you have the power to do so.

CHAPTER 13

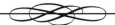

Choices

I T'S BEEN MY GOAL TO make you aware that you have choices other than conventional or traditional medicine, lots of them, and we've been led to believe by all the fear and propaganda out there that we don't. We've been led to believe the medical profession doesn't know what causes cancer or how to cure it and that cancer and other diseases have little or nothing to do with nutrition. That's a lot of boloney! Maybe they refuse to focus on the easy way to cure things because their egos won't let them digest the fact that, yes, it can be as simple as the food, air, and water we put into our bodies as well as the belief systems we live by. We do have a choice, the cures are out there, and I want you and the whole world to know about them.

I recently was talking to a friend who went home to visit his mother and sisters only to find out that both of his sisters within two weeks of each other had been diagnosed with breast cancer. One was a false alarm, but the other sister did indeed have breast cancer. After talking with her husband of over thirty years and her family, the sister who had the malignancy decided to have a complete mastectomy, both breasts. My heart just sank when I heard this. As a woman I couldn't imagine losing that part of my femininity.

Think about this: Was it her breasts that caused her to experience breast cancer? No, it was not her breasts. Her breasts are where her malfunctioning immune system showed up. Yet the medical doctors offered her a mastectomy as part of the treatment, along with possibly some radiation and chemotherapy. Did they tell her they *got it all* with the breast removal? What does *got it all* mean, anyway? Maybe they saw no more cancer cells in the tissue samples, but they sure as heck didn't get to what caused her cancer. Did they discuss the intricacies of her diet and how a body's cells are affected by the different foods we eat? Probably not. They didn't get it all. All they did was mutilate her unnecessarily. What caused her to get cancer? Surely not having breasts. This is just so wrong.

Fear is incredibly toxic, and until we have all the information about our choices, this kind of mutilation will continue by medical doctors who do not know or understand the power of plants and other forms of alternative applications and solutions.

You can't put eleven ounces of water in a ten-ounce glass without it spilling out. You can't put ten pounds of potatoes in a five-pound sack, and you can't put excessive amounts of fat, sugar, alcohol, poisonous prescription drugs, and lifeless processed foods into your body without harm. You can't do these things without serious consequences or an internal health revolt. It becomes a case of toxins versus healthy organs and other intricate systems. There are more bad guys than good guys when disease sets in. There are more troops in the toxic camp than there are in the healthy camp. That's what happens when your body is full of toxicity; it spills out in the form of sickness and disease. Your body starts an internal battle with itself. Your body just can't fight it any longer. Changing your eating habits is an inside job. It has to start with you and an ultimate desire to want incredible health and to want to stay that way.

Yes, you do have a choice. You especially have a choice in the case of deciding to use traditional medicine or alternatives, or even a combination of the two. Each case requires separate evaluation. There is no one size fits all. These systems are no longer mutually exclusive and can work well together as a team. The medical profession must acknowledge, apply and assist their patients with understanding the power of rebuilding the immune system using a plant based diet, detoxifying the body from harsh chemicals and poisons, the power of using natural vitamin and mineral supplements and the power of positive belief systems.

It's not impossible. It's really, "I'm-possible." If we ultimately want the best health for the whole planet, it starts with one. That one is you; that one is me; that one is your neighbor. Together we make up the planet; together we make up the world. What kind of world will it be?

So *stop it!* Stop all those bad habits, one at a time, little by little. You can do it. Start doing some of your own research to explore the things you feel need the most attention and get going. Your vibrant life is waiting for you!

The following poem was delivered to me in just five minutes by my guardian angels the day after I thought I had finished writing this book. This poem, "Note to My Soul," is a summary and in harmony with what this message is all about. I hope you enjoy it.

Note to My Soul

Dear God,
As I lay this book to rest,
I vow to do my very best.
In the raw, or in the nude,
I'll try to find the right attitude.

I'll treat my body with respect.
The drugs and toxins I have left.
I'll fill it with a rainbow of colors
That will nourish and replenish.

Let go of fear, you bet I will.
A bounty of love awaits my fill.
My life is mine, for me to choose,
As no one else can wear my shoes.

I am you,
And you are me.
When once I know this,
I'll be free.

I am ready.
I am going
To embark on this journey
And find my new flowing.

The peace and tranquility
That I will find
Will forever release me
From the unbalanced grind.

I love me, I love me, I love me, I do.
Only now
Do I know
I can love all of you too!

Namaste!

Chapter 14

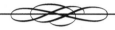

Testimonials

Jim Miller
A Cancer Death Sentence
I Don't Think So!

miller@lake-real-estate.com
352-504-0070

In September 2006, Mandy, my massage therapist, told me that my spleen was like a rock and I better get it checked out. In November, when I finally went to Dr. Taylor, he informed me that my hemoglobin was at 6 and it should be between 12 and16 and was ordering two units of blood for me at Waterman Hospital. He was pretty sure I had cancer in my bone marrow, which was inhibiting my production of red blood cells. He said they could stave it off with chemo, but it would keep coming back faster and faster until they couldn't do any more chemo, and then I would die maybe in five to ten years.

He referred me to Dr. Tumala, who is a wonderful oncologist, to get a full diagnosis.

Dr. Tumala did a bone marrow biopsy and ordered a PET scan. He told me that I had Non-Hodgkin's Leukemic Lymphoma (NHLL), proving Dr.

Taylor's suspicion. I started chemo in January 2007. I did six cycles—four weeks apart—eight hours on Monday followed by two hours on Tuesday and Wednesday. I finished in June 2007, and Dr. Tumala did a bone marrow biopsy and ordered a PET scan again. The chemo worked. My spleen was soft, and my biopsy results showed that I was in full remission, but a new – not as aggressive – strain of cancer showed up that was at 6-7 percent.

Because NHLL always comes back, Dr. Tumala suggested that I consider a bone-marrow transplant and referred me to Moffitt Cancer Center in Tampa, Florida, where I met with the acknowledged expert in the field. He was upbeat because they were now 60-70 percent successful. Success was defined as living five years—not a cure. So they were going to almost poison me to death to kill my bone marrow and my immune system (so I wouldn't reject the donor marrow) while damaging many organs in the hope that I might survive and live five years.

That is when I chose to look at my sister-in-law's suggestion that I try Hippocrates Health Institute in West Palm Beach, Florida. It couldn't hurt, and it might work. I could always take my chances with the bone-marrow transplant later. Just before I left for Hippocrates, Mandy told me that my spleen was getting lumpy again. Dr. Tumala was right, the NHLL was coming back. I didn't tell my wife.

I arrived at Hippocrates the Sunday before Thanksgiving 2007 and stayed for three weeks. It was a wonderful place, and it worked! When I got back Mandy couldn't find my spleen; it was completely soft. My blood counts were improving. In June 2008, Dr. Tumala did a bone marrow biopsy and ordered a PET scan. Again, I was in full remission (last November we knew the NHLL had come back because of my lumpy spleen) and the strain that was 6-7 percent was now 0.1 percent. Since then my blood counts have continued to be low but stable. Dr. Tumala now checks me every sixty days instead of every thirty days. More importantly, I feel great! I just turned sixty and feel better than I did at thirty. I have boundless energy, and people keep telling me how good I look.

In some ways cancer may have been a blessing because I never would have gone to Hippocrates if I had not been offered a bone-marrow transplant. They have an expression at Hippocrates, "You are here because you are enlightened or you are frightened."

I was frightened. But because of my new lifestyle, I feel my next sixty years will be better than the first sixty years.

What Is the Lifestyle That Has Transformed My Life?
Alternative to Cancer Death Sentence

Hippocrates is an oasis for healing all diseases—diabetes, cancer, etc. Their three-week program helps you focus on your mind, body, and spirit. Besides their wonderful diet they have lectures and exercise classes all day long. We were taught that exercise and sleep are essential to health and healing, as is peace of mind and joy. They even brought in a doctor who taught us laughter therapy. Laughter (even if you don't feel like it) is very therapeutic.

When I arrived at Hippocrates Health Institute, I weighed 216 pounds and was frightened, but determined. I have weighed as much as 256 pounds. Today I weigh 156 pounds. While there, I lost 21 pounds during the three weeks and was never hungry, nor did I crave anything.

The main thing they do (and I still do) is every morning and afternoon drink sixteen ounces of fresh, green juice made out of sprouts (sunflower is the most nutritious and powerful), cucumber, and celery; plus two to three ounces of wheatgrass juice separately. Wheatgrass is very cleansing and a strong anti-cancer agent, as is raw garlic. I add a clove of garlic to my juice every time.

Except for Wednesdays, we had lunch and dinner buffets of raw vegetables and vegetable dishes. Raw food is alive, but when you heat it over 118 degrees you scramble the enzymes; if you microwave it, you totally wreck it. The food was good, but I could barely eat a plateful in thirty minutes, as they taught us to chew our food until it was puree before swallowing. I used to clean my plate in five minutes, tops. On Wednesdays we fasted, doing only the juices. I was never hungry.

My body was getting all the nutrients it needed. It was getting whole, live food, not the processed, cooked diet that I had grown to love. I am now totally vegan. That means I eat no meats, cheese, or eggs. People ask,

"What do you do for protein?" Have you ever seen a horse or a bull? What do they do for protein? Animal protein is way overrated (especially by the dairy and meat industries); mother's milk is 90 percent carbohydrates, 5 percent protein, and 5 percent fatty acids—and we double our size in the first year.

I was taught that cancer thrives in a low-oxygen, acidic environment. Therefore, I can't have fruit or starches like corn, etc. because they have sugar, which takes the oxygen out of my blood. I can't have carrots or even beets, as they both have a high sugar content. The "American diet," with meat, dairy, and fried and processed foods, is very acidic.

I learned to focus on what I can eat—lots of delicious raw-food dishes— not what I can't eat. TV commercials can be a little disconcerting. In my old life I ate to feel good; now I feel good because of what I eat. They taught us "It's not the food in your life, but the life in your food!"

They also stressed a clean colon. We carry lots of old and toxic waste in our colon. John Wayne had over fifty pounds in his colon when he died. We gave ourselves enemas daily, and we received a colonic every week we were there. That explains some of my weight loss. I go back quarterly for the pools and a colonic. When I graduated, I stated, "It was an honor to graduate with honors from Enema University." I received some understanding laughs.

Feel free to e-mail me questions at miller@lake-real-estate.com or check out Hippocrates at www.HippocratesInst.org. One could "do Hippocrates" on a budget by purchasing their DVDs, but if you have a serious health issue, it is best to do the three weeks.

If you don't do e-mail, I can be reached at 352-504-0070.

Written Saturday, August 8, 2009 by Jim Miller

As of June 1, 2010, I have no symptoms of cancer whatsoever. My blood counts are normal, and everyone tells me how "good" I look at 183lbs. I now eat cooked food and fruit, but still 100 percent vegan (no meat, dairy or eggs), avoiding flour, sugar, potatoes, soda, alcohol, and coffee.

Shirley A. Snyder

Knowing I was very ill and dying, I saw fifteen doctors in Florida, but not one of them could tell me what was wrong with me. That experience itself should be published. Finally, my dermatologist told me I was very ill and made an appointment with a doctor friend of his who put me in the hospital and did a battery of tests. They found a tumor in my colon that was previously missed. I went to Michigan to a family friend who happened to be a cancer surgeon. He told me I had colon cancer and opened me up to find I also had a metastasized liver. He told my family I had weeks to live and told me I was too weak (eighty-nine pounds) for chemo and radiation, and there was nothing he knew that I could do to save myself.

I am an Aries, and we do not give up. Being a paralegal I decided to do some research and found alternative medicine. Off to the health store I went. In 1988 I thought there were some very weird people and unfamiliar products there because, although I ate in some very fine restaurants, I also ate junk food and prepared food, smoked, and loved good wine and Diet Pepsi. Also, my job was very stressful and caused me to work long hours. Yes, I do know exactly what caused the cancer.

Soon I became one of those weird people in the health-food stores. I quit smoking, gave up alcohol, ate only organic products, and gave up sugar altogether once I learned that sugar feeds cancer. My mother would buy free-range chickens and make soup. It took me a year to get on my feet, but I never doubted that I could get well. I studied alternative medicine and vibrational energy relentlessly.

I have been cancer-free for twenty-one years. I graduated from the Global College of Natural Medicine and have certificates as a Holistic Practitioner, Nutritional Consultant, and Master Herbalist. I do not practice because I am not licensed and because I promised myself if I could get well I would help anyone interested in knowing how I beat cancer. My friends call me a walking encyclopedia on the subject of alternative health, but I do not let it overpower my life, although going to an organic farmer's market is my favorite thing to do.

My journey should be a book of its own because I cannot cover in a few paragraphs all the knowledge I was fortunate enough to experience.

Phil Hartten

419 504 9450

phil@hartten.com

Cancer, yes, I had it three times now. It is gone. I don't take any meds and defy illness. If germs enter, my instructions are to kill the germs instantly and completely. I am in charge now.

Someone asked me, "Where is the immune system in your body?"

I said it is in my brain, a very powerful weapon indeed. I have to feed my brain properly with nutrition. The universe supplies the unlimited knowledge that is needed, and I receive and implement it.

Be sure to understand that we have to do our part daily. Nutrition, exercise, and restraint go together. Determine your body type and nutrition needs by reading *Perfect Health* written by Deepak Chopra. Then do it. Every day do your job. It is not about what I want. It is all about what my body needs to stay healthy. There is "no cake and eat it too."

Watch people who are overweight and do not exercise as they should. The nursing homes are full and waiting for the next guy or gal who refuses to live life under life's terms. It is not by my terms that I live now. We must do our part, and do it daily.

Learn about what your brain takes as food. Learn to receive and believe. We are like the Christmas tree that is all decorated but not plugged in. We need to get plugged in, and then we will have the glow of health and be lean and strong.

Analyze just what your core values are and what you really believe. Is your door of belief only partially open? Throw it wide open and receive your full share of spiritual healing, abundance, contentment, and caring.

We all are incredibly huge believers, yet we deny it. Think about the red light when driving. You stop, every time. It is your belief that if you do not, bad things can and may occur. You believe every day that water is always wet, the tides will change periodically, and gravity will hold you down. You are a big believer already, so use your beliefs and expand them fully. Get your healing and quit the meds and crazy testing.

Joy Matwyshen

My name is Joy Matwyshen, and I have been an organic gardener for thirty-nine years. It was a critical illness that led me to make this choice and to live a natural and organic lifestyle so that my body could detoxify and heal itself.

I became very sick in my early twenties with kidney and bladder problems. Before I knew it, taking medication became a way of life. One of the symptoms I experienced was blood in my urine with lots of pain. The side effects went from one new health issue to another. I found myself getting sicker and sicker, weaker and weaker, with little or no energy all of the time.

After going from bad to worse over a period of three years, I was diagnosed with chronic kidney disease and told that it was irreversible; the next step would be dialysis. This was a bombshell for me. The waiting lines were long for kidney dialysis, and without dialysis life expectancy is no longer than a year or two. I knew I was in bad shape because, at that point, I had no quality of life. When I would walk down the hall from the bedroom to the kitchen many times I had to hold onto the wall because everything would get black and I would almost pass out. I was taking handsful of prescription medications that affected my sinuses, breathing, and mental clarity. My head, nose, and ears felt all plugged up; I was miserable because I felt horrible.

I was given a book titled *How To Get Well* by Paavo Airola, N.D., that gave me hope and direction. Dr. Airola basically explained that a lifestyle of not feeding your body real nutrition and overexposure to toxic chemicals (including medications) slows down the glandular and metabolic rate, and the eliminative organs lose their efficiency. That made sense to me! Through my childhood I had been exposed to chemicals being sprayed on the fields while we were picking vegetables. We even chased after the mosquito spraying clouds, not knowing any of that was potentially harmful to us or that anything toxic was building up in our bodies. We were given antibiotics every time we had the flu. Couple that with years of a typical American diet of meat, dairy, lots of processed and chemically-raised foods (never anything grown organically), toss in some stress, and there you have a "toxic" lifestyle that created a lot of toxicity throughout my body.

Dr. Airola explained that "you must change your lifestyle in order to gain maximum, vibrant health." I knew this was something I had to do! I decided to stop the medications that I knew were not helping me and made me feel horrible. I stopped eating a toxic diet and began juicing with 100 percent organic raw vegetables. I understood from the book that I may feel worse at first while my body dumped all of those toxins. I'm glad I knew that, because I really felt worse to begin with as I went through a healing crisis. After the third week I began to see a great change in my energy and how I felt.

Within three months I felt like a different person. I knew I was on my way to living a vibrant life! I followed my organic, raw-vegetable juicing and blending for nearly one year. It not only gave me my life back, but I became vibrantly healthy for the first time in my life. Then I started adding 100 percent organic raw and living foods (soaked and sprouted seeds, nuts, grains, legumes, and berries), along with my freshly made juices, to my lifestyle. Eventually, I added lightly steamed/cooked vegetables. I also started learning how to live a stress-free, worry-free, fear-free life, which is a very important part of establishing and maintaining vibrant health.

My son's babysitter introduced me to organic gardening and helped me prepare my first organic garden in 1974. She was also the one who introduced me to Ira Ebersole. The radical change that came about in my health in a relatively short time was phenomenal. I hate to think where I would be today at age sixty-four if I had not made that change; it has continued to be my lifestyle for thirty-nine years.

Today I feel vibrant and full of energy, and do not get sick. I stay away from processed and commercially grown foods as much as I possibly can. We were not created from chemicals; neither can we sustain life with them. I learned so much over the years, and I have a passion to help others who are striving to live a vibrant, healthy life—free from sickness, disease, worry, stress, poverty, and anything else that robs them of enjoying the abundant life our creator desires us to have! That is why "Seed Time to Harvest" was birthed, and that is why "Seed Time to Harvest" is dedicated to helping others live a healthy and vibrant life!

Jean Sumner

Being diagnosed with cancer was the best thing that ever happened to me. Let me tell you what I mean by that statement.

My story begins on May 9, 2009, when I met with an oncologist, and she told me I had cancer. The interesting thing about the diagnosis was that the cancer I had was incurable according to the medical world. I recall asking the oncologist if lifestyle and diet could make a difference, and she answered this question with an astounding *no*! Can you believe it? Diet and lifestyle always make a difference! Prior to this diagnosis I lived what the mainstream world would consider a very healthy life. I exercised at least five days a week, ate according to the food pyramid, avoided red meat, ate lots of salads, watched the type of fat that I used, and ate very little sugar. Needless to say a diagnosis of cancer was very shocking. I do have to tell you that I was definitely a Type A personality.

But wait, I am not the type of person to let someone put an expiration stamp on my life. Fortunately for me, I had met Lynn (the person who would become my spiritual coach) a couple of years earlier and bumped into her a day before I was to see the doctor for the test results. Talk about synchronicity! When I saw her I told her that I might need to meet with her. Now you must realize that I had no idea what Lynn did. Along with this step I found a book called *The Cancer Battle Plan* by David and Anne Frahm. Anne had breast cancer; she had had chemo twice, radiation twice, and two surgeries when the doctors sent her home to die. In the book she talks about changing her diet to vegetarian, drinking essiac tea, and consuming a green drink called Kyogreen. She lived another six or seven years and eventually died from the effects of her cancer treatment. So I changed my diet to vegetarian, purchased Kyogreen, and called Lynn.

One thing you should know about me is that my training was in accounting and I had spent twenty-seven years being a commercial banker. I was very left-brained and proud of my great logic. My first session with Lynn was just weird! But something kept me coming back for more sessions.

During this time I continued to do research and learn more and more about possible ways to get rid of the cancer. The next step in my catharsis was meeting Jim Miller, who was diagnosed with non-Hodgkin's lymphoma. He had one bout of chemo, and the cancer came back in three months in a very aggressive form. The doctors wanted to do a bone marrow transplant. Fortunately for Jim, he knew someone who guided him to Hippocrates Health Center in West Palm Beach, Florida. At Hippocrates Jim learned how to eat a raw-food diet. They also had many colonics to clean out the digestive system, and they worked on spirituality. Two years later, Jim was cancer-free. After learning his story I decided to make some more changes. I started to eat raw. This was an interesting and difficult change. It required a new recipe for every meal. I also started getting a weekly massage and visiting a chiropractor on a regular basis. And it was about this time that I purchased an infrared sauna, which I began using daily. Everything that I was doing was taking an enormous amount of time, and along with trying to be well, I was working as a commercial banker on a fulltime basis. It was very difficult. But I was determined not to worry about that date stamp the doctors had given me.

It was about this time that I was sitting in a Rotary meeting listening to a speaker talk about the impact Rotary has had on his life. His speech was so compelling that I had tears running down my face. At that moment I decided I wanted to do something in my life that I could be as passionate about as the speaker was about Rotary. And I knew it wasn't Rotary. I decided to start clubs similar to Rotary but with a focus on wellness. Now here is another moment where I was definitely guided. I called a woman that I had met only twice and told her of my idea. Between the two of us we started World Wellness Education, a nonprofit organization whose mission is to educate the world about wellness one story at a time. Our focus was on mind, body, and spirit, with an emphasis on people sharing their healing stories. We started with clubs, and now we have a TV show, conference calls on the Internet, and a radio show, with each of these venues focusing on a healing story.

During this time I continued to have sessions with Lynn. She would give me CDs to listen to that were changing my entire belief system. And it seemed that people continued to enter my life who were more spiritual, and they continued to provide me with more information about books to read, movies to watch, and CDs to listen to about spirituality. I learned to meditate, and Lynn gave me great CDs to facilitate my meditation.

Of course I continued to scour the Internet for anyone who had cured the type of cancer with which I had been diagnosed. Finally I found one story about an individual in Australia who had brought his test numbers back into the normal range by having all of his dental fillings removed. So now I had a new mission. In January 2010 I had about 50 percent of the silver fillings removed from my mouth. Due to insurance limitations, I had to wait until January 2011, to complete the process. In this time I learned a lot about the toxic effect of "silver fillings," and my mouth was full of them. I remember one dental appointment as a teenager where I was given thirteen fillings at one time. It is quite funny that the world of dentistry calls them "silver fillings," considering they are 50 percent mercury. Studies reveal that mercury causes brain damage in children, Alzheimer's disease, neurological problems, and gastrointestinal problems.

Now I have to tell you that all of the things I had changed were not making a difference. Every three months I would have a blood test, and I would anxiously await the results, only to find that the numbers had increased. Meanwhile, I had never felt better in my life. My skin glowed from the great diet, I had lost all my excess weight, and everyone I saw would tell me how great I looked.

I started to engage more with Lynn and her groups. Along with weekly sessions with Lynn, I started to meet with her group on a regular basis. They were really expanding my mind and sometimes blowing my mind. We were studying Atlantis, The Essene Teachings, Drunvalo Melchizedek,

Crystal Energy, Auras, etc. With all of this my spirituality began to bloom, and I continued to change.

In the fall of 2010 I became extremely exhausted. I was falling asleep driving my car— not a good idea! This was one symptom of the cancer. That is about the time I heard about a doctor who uses oxygen therapy to cure cancer. She actually combined oxygen and saline solution and gave it to me intravenously. I followed this course of treatment for about nine months. In the spring of 2011, after six months of oxygen treatment, two years of changing my diet, expanding my spirituality, learning to relax, and three months after getting all of the "silver fillings" out of my mouth, my numbers started coming down. When I was first diagnosed my white blood count was 13,000. Over time it rose to 19,000 and my last blood test had the white blood count down to 13,000 again.

So when I say being diagnosed with cancer was the best thing that has ever happened in my life, it is easy to see why. It completely changed my life. Without this diagnosis I would never have experienced the level of spirituality that I experience today, World Wellness Education would never have come about, and I would never have enjoyed the benefits of truly eating well because I was using the assumption that the government food pyramid had some basis in fact. How was one to know that it had a basis in money, not health? I would never have enjoyed working in a field where I have such passion. I would never have learned the joy and benefits of meditation. And the list goes on.

Today I look at my diagnosis as God's way of nudging me in the direction that I was supposed to be moving my whole life!

Heidi Buffett
How Cancer Gave Me Health and a Wealth of Knowledge

My cancer journey started in July, 2003. My bags were packed for a trip to Europe to go to a wedding near Vienna, Austria, and then visit relatives throughout Germany. I just had a routine mammogram, and the day before my flight, I got a call from my doctor's office to come in right away. He told me that I had breast cancer. He said that they needed to do a biopsy right away and then do surgery. It was a shock to hear that, but I didn't get too upset because the cancer diagnosis didn't really sink in. All I could think of was not being able to go to the wedding and, more importantly, that I didn't get any trip cancellation insurance. I had booked the $1,200 flight only a week earlier, and nothing was going to happen within a week, right? Wrong! Everything can change in an instant, and I should have been the one to know better, because not too long before that, my husband gave me a hug and then several minutes later fell over and died instantly of a heart attack. Could the stress of losing him have brought on my cancer? Or could it have been the "healthy" foods that I was eating? At least I thought that I was eating a healthy diet. On top of that, I never smoked, never drank any alcohol, and I was always trying to stay fit by exercising.

So I had the biopsy. Then I had the surgery. Then I was sent to see an oncologist. He told me that they needed to start me on chemo right away, and then I would need to have thirty-six radiation treatments. There had never been any cancer diagnosis to any of my family members, so I didn't really know too much about it. I did everything that all my doctors and specialists had told me to.

After I was driven home from the first chemo treatment, I got so sick and kept vomiting. After the third treatment, I lost all my hair. On top of the constant vomiting, I developed blisters in my mouth, my gums were sore, my teeth were weakening, and I lost my sense of taste.

Being so sick and all alone at home, I had reached the point where I didn't want to continue with this, and I didn't care if I ever woke up again. I had even thought to myself that maybe this is my late husband's way of getting me to join him.

Then one day my son, Michael, and his wife, Kelly, dropped by to see me. They handed me a bag and said, "This is a little gift to make you feel better."

I looked inside and pulled out a bib that said "I love grandma" on it. I looked at it for a while, and then they realized that I was very confused and did not really know what this bib was for. (I later learned this condition was called "chemo brain.") So my son told me that Kelly was pregnant.

After they left, and thinking about it some more, it finally dawned on me that I was going to be a grandmother to my first grandchild. Now I had to rethink everything—I needed to survive this cancer. I had to get better in order to see my first grandchild.

Sometime shortly thereafter I got a phone call from my mother, telling me about this Chinese naturopathic doctor who had helped a lot of cancer patients. I got an appointment with him, and he told me that we needed to build up my immune system and rebuild all the good cells that had now been destroyed by the chemo. He proceeded to put a bunch of herbs into a bowl. Then he put these herbs into a machine, which then made tea bags out of them. I was to drink this tea numerous times a day. He also told me to stop eating meat, white sugar, (cancer cells thrive on sugar), white flour, and dairy. By the time I left his office, I walked out with a large bag full of herbal supplements, teas, and natural vitamins.

When I mentioned this to my oncologist, he did not want me to take anything other than what he prescribed (chemical drugs). The Chinese naturopathic doctor had told me that none of the "natural" products would interfere with my chemo. They would only be of benefit to my body. So I continued taking what this Chinese doctor recommended for me, without saying anymore to my oncologist.

It wasn't long after that when I started feeling a bit better. I wasn't as nauseated, and my blood count was up again.

After my treatments were finished, I decided that I was now on a mission—to get my health to the best state that it has ever been and to live a healthy, disease-free, energetic life. "Wealth" was no longer at the top of my priority list. I have now replaced that with "health."

I started taking numerous classes on health and nutrition, as well as courses on vegan and raw foods. I even took several courses with Deepak Chopra. One of them was about *ayurveda* and food as medicine, and the other course was on meditation.

From all my research and the courses I've taken, I have come to the conclusion that we are living in a toxic world and that almost all health problems stem from a western "dead" food diet. *Look no further than*

216

what's on your plate. The foods you're eating are making you fat, robbing your energy, and killing your body.

Besides being a raw-vegan, I am now learning how to live off the land. Those weeds that you're all trying to kill—they are the healthiest and most powerful food and medicine on the planet. For almost every health condition you face, nature offers a safe and effective remedy. "Weeds" have amazing healing qualities, and best of all, they're *free*! Nature and wild plants give us enough food and healing power to never get sick again. *Eat your weeds*!

In conclusion, I must add that since my recovery from cancer, and after gaining a wealth of knowledge, I have never been sick (not even a cold). I have more energy at sixty-two years of age than I did in my twenties. I've lost almost twenty-five pounds. I've cured my sleep apnea, and my vision has improved. I am continually striving to gain more knowledge and more health. It's a whole lifestyle change!

Bill Kingsley
My Coronary Artery Miracle

It was an early Friday afternoon at my cardiologist's office when he suggested it was probably time for a heart catheterization, and I agreed. He made a call, and I had an early morning appointment for the following Tuesday. A few months earlier I had a complete workup—EKG, Nuclear Stress Test, etc. I did not do so well, and he suggested medications—blood thinners and statin drugs, which I have used previously and which I resisted because of their side effects and my doubts about their efficacy.

I came to his office that Friday because for the past year or so I had experienced angina when I exercised, bicycled, and walked, and during a trip to Colorado, with elevations of over 7,000 feet, I really felt stressed, a clear sign of arterial blockage.

I have had a history of high cholesterol and was diagnosed with coronary-artery disease. Sixteen years ago at the age of sixty-three I had successful triple-bypass surgery. Sixteen years is a long time without a recurrence of arterial re-clogging; hence, my visit to the doctor.

I Gave Myself Cancer, I Can Take It Away!

Twenty years or so ago, after I had become disenchanted with western religions, I began a spiritual journey for knowledge of self, soul, and life's meaning. I have read many philosophies and, simply put, I came to an understanding that everything is in vibration and connected and that "thoughts are things."

The week that my doctor made a surgery appointment for me, I was watching a new DVD by one of my teachers, Dr. Wayne Dyer, as he was relating some Bible and real-life stories to the audience.

I understood that we are all connected, and that I am a part of God, as a drop of water is of the ocean—that, as God, we can heal ourselves. I am that I am.

That Friday night, as I was falling asleep, all of that went through my mind, and I began to realize, to know, that I was able to heal myself and that my arteries were experiencing a cleansing. I felt the healing. Periodically over the rest of the weekend, I experienced that same feeling of cleansing, and I had a knowing that when I went for surgery on Tuesday, the surgeon would not find any blockages.

Come Tuesday morning, en route to the hospital, a moment of doubt flashed through my mind, and I thought that maybe the surgeon would find one clogged artery. I immediately switched that thought and remembered from Dr. Dyer's message, "banish all doubt."

I had to wait in pre-op for a few hours before my turn in the cath lab. I met the doctor who would perform the procedure; he related that he had performed over 30,000 of these procedures. I was soon rolled into the O.R., prepped, and the next thing I remember I was waking up. The doctor said I was clean, that he did not need to use any stents, and all my arteries were clear.

In the recovery room he told me my grafts from sixteen years ago looked great and gave me a copy of my coronary tree that was generated from the monitor he used during the surgery. The only blockages were those that had been bypassed so many years ago. He said my arteries and grafts looked great and that I could resume exercise.

That I have done. I continue to ride my bike, walk, and play racket sports (pickle ball). No more angina or shortness of breath. On a follow-up with my cardiologist, he said to come back in a year. I have released all doubts.

Carol Lynch
Osteoporosis to Osteopenia Solution

March 29, 2011

Yes, I had osteoporosis five years ago. I was devastated when I got the results from my first bone-density test in The Villages. I had a 30 percent bone loss in my left hip. Wow, how could this happen to me? I knew I had bone loss from tests I had while living in Boston, but this was a shock.

God was on my side because I just happened to call my friend, Joanne. She told me about her friend who used to have osteoporosis and no longer did. How could this be? Once you have it, you have it forever. Not true. I called her friend, and she told me that if I did what she told me to do I would also get rid of my osteoporosis.

One year later I had another bone density test, this time with another doctor. I changed doctors because the first doctor wanted me to take Fosamax. My daughter, who was studying to be a nutritionist, told me not to take it because of all the side effects. This second doctor said, "Mrs. Lynch, I'm so sorry to tell you that you have 15 percent bone loss in your left hip." I was so excited that I jumped all over the place. He couldn't believe it when I told him that just one year ago I had 30 percent bone loss in that same hip.

If you do what I suggest, you, too, can get rid of your osteoporosis. There are no side effects; it's all natural and inexpensive. A product called Ultimate Bone Builder by Ethical Nutrients contains glucosamine sulfate and ipriflavone. There are quite a few bone builders on the market, but this is the one that does the trick. The reason it's so effective is that it contains a substance called microcrystalline hydroxyapatite, which helps to build bones. I take six tablets every day, two after each meal, with a large glass of water. It works; I'm living proof. It was also suggested that I take a quality multivitamin that contains vitamin D and zinc. I've been doing this now for almost five years, and I now have osteopenia, which is a great improvement over osteoporosis.

Bone-building exercises are important; I walk and lift weights every single day. I even had a doctor write down the information for her mother! Imagine that! A medical doctor *asking her patient for information on how to heal*!

Magnesium
I Feel Young Again
Antoine

As a young boy growing up and even into adulthood I experienced a lot of stress involving family, religious and work related situations. It seems I never slept more than a couple of hours straight because my mind was always reeling about something. I couldn't turn it off. Afternoon naps were unavoidable. The pure exhaustion was exasperating and I literally slept at my job after lunch sitting upright in my chair.

A friend of mine sent me an Internet link to some information on the importance of magnesium in your diet and the side effects which could be experienced for someone seriously deficient in this important mineral.

I looked at these side effects and realized I had ALL of them, all at the same time to one degree or another. I thought; *let's give it a try, what have I got to lose*? I bought some and in just a few days all of my symptoms literally disappeared. This is not an exaggeration, they all quite literally vanished. My muscle spasms, irregular heartbeat, chest pains are all gone. I now sleep, uninterrupted, through the night without night sweats or aches and pains. Even after extended lawn and yard work I don't experience any muscle soreness or fatigue.

I used to get sinus headaches all the time. A doctor told me that acid reflux was the cause of the sinus headaches and all he prescribed was the usual prescription antacids which did in fact seem to help for the last twelve years. However after taking daily magnesium supplements, my acid riddled stomach and sinus headaches are now gone.

Here are some of the symptoms that I was suffering from:

- Aches and pains
- Fatigue
- Poor digestion
- Blood sugar imbalance
- Poor sleep
- Muscle twitching and or cramps
- Short term memory gaps
- Chest pain
- Headaches
- Irregular heartbeat

It's just plain amazing how doctors don't recommend natural cures. Seriously, twelve years of Ranitidine? When you get a diagnosis of any kind and your doctor prescribes a pharmaceutical drug, just ask if there is some natural supplement that could replace the drug. If the doctor insists on the drug, then getting a second and third opinion may be the way to go.

This works so well, I told everyone I know. By taking magnesium, my dad, a border line diabetic, lowered his blood sugar level. My English friend and her whole family now take magnesium too. It's a bit funny. One of the grand kids came up to my friend and asked, "What the bloody hell are you giving my Nan (Grand Mom)? ...She's acting younger than me!"

I'm now in my late forties and so grateful I've found a natural remedy, a natural cure that is easy to take, without side effects and gives me so much relief I no longer feel old. I feel young and love life again.

APPENDIX A

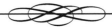

Growing Wheatgrass and Sunflower Sprouts

Trays

4 – 11"x 24"x 2" plastic trays with holes for drainage

Amount of Seeds per Tray

1½ cups of wheatgrass for each tray of wheatgrass you will be growing

2 cups of sunnies (sunflower seeds) per tray

Soaking

Soak seeds in separate bowls overnight.

Add enough water until it is an inch above the top of the seeds.

Sunflower seeds float, that's OK.

Next Day

Drain seeds in a colander all day and rinse once or twice during the day, if you can.

Use a mesh strainer to prevent the seeds from falling through the bottom of regular pasta strainers.

Planting

Put in enough topsoil or potting soil so that it compacts to about ½" deep in each tray.

Compact the soil with an empty tray.

Plant sunflower seeds and wheatgrass seeds in separate trays.

Spread the seeds out evenly over the topsoil.

Water, then cover the planted wheatgrass trays and sunflower trays with another empty tray to simulate being in the ground.

It's a good idea to plant sunnies and wheatgrass at the same time so you can use the wheatgrass tray to put on top of the planted sunnies until the sunnies reach the top level of the planting tray.

Wheatgrass

In two to three days the wheatgrass will grow to be at the top level of the planting tray. You can now remove the top tray and leave it off for the growing duration.

Sunnies

Sunnies need the extra weight of a planted tray of wheatgrass on top of them in order to simulate pushing through soil.

When the sunnies reach the top edge of the planting tray, about three to four days, you can remove the empty tray and the planted wheatgrass tray.

Don't store your empty trays under a planted tray of either wheatgrass or sunnies as this could create a moisture problem and encourage mold growth.

Where to Grow

If you own your own home you can use your garage to start the growing process.

If you live in a condo or villa without a garage, you can begin the process in the bathtub. Use very low light during the day and turn off the light at night. (I live on the third floor of a condo building without a garage and I use my spare bathtub. It works great.) Once the sunnies and wheatgrass reach the top level of the planting trays, I move them to a sunny area in my kitchen to get some bright sunlight during the day and bring them back to the bathtub in the evening for watering and draining.

I experimented with allowing them to grow full time in the bathtub versus bringing them into the sunlight during the day. I found giving the sunnies and wheatgrass sunlight during the day caused them to grow faster and much greener. For me this created a more tolerable wheatgrass juice rather than let it grow under dim light in the bathtub where it never got quite as green. The sunnies got taller in the bathtub but not as green.

Watering

If you have chlorinated water, fill your watering can and let it sit overnight to cause most, if not all, of the chlorine to dissipate. Do this every night so you're watering with de-chlorinated water the next day.

Take the empty trays off both the planted wheatgrass trays and sunnie trays only to water during the first few days. Also take the planted wheatgrass trays off sunnies only to water.

Water every night. Just soak them—no need to over water as this may cause mold.

Each environment is different. Water less if you have a humid area, more if it's drier.

You just have to experiment and see what works best for you.

Don't forget to put the planted wheatgrass trays back on top of the sunnies.

Toward the last few days of growing the sunnies may need more water.

Low Light

No direct sunlight during the first few days.

Just enough to see; one small wattage light bulb is plenty.

Wheatgrass and sunnies will not sprout in bright light.

Turn the light off at night and back on in the morning.

Bring your sunnies and wheatgrass into a partly sunny or sunny area of your home during the day after they reach to top edge of the growing tray.

Watch Them Grow

Once the sunnies have pushed the wheatgrass tray as high as the top edge of the sunnie tray, leave them uncovered until harvest.

Harvest

Harvest just before the grass (about seven days) and sunnies (about ten days) "split."

After the grass and the sunnies split, meaning they produce another pair of leaves, they become adult plants and lose much of the nutritional value they have as tender babies.

The longer you wait to harvest the sunnies, the fewer hulls will be present, but again harvest before they begin to grow a second pair of leaves.

Some mold may occur; this is quite normal.

Use a good, sharp pair of scissors or a knife and cut the plants just above the mold, if any.

Store in gallon sized plastic storage bags or some other container of your choice.

Important

It's best not to re-use the root system of the harvested wheatgrass and sunnies again because you will never have the same nutritional value as with the first growing.

Topsoil is cheap, so discard or compost the old root system and start over again.

When washing the trays, be sure to wash both sides to prevent mold from growing.

A small fan moving the air around may inhibit mold if you're using your garage to grow these.

YouTube link to Jim Miller's thirty-minute wheatgrass growing video.
http://www.youtube.com/watch?v=R1ysca2lidI

Sunflower Sprouts

Thirty times more nutritious than broccoli

Wheatgrass Juice

Loaded with antioxidants.

Wheatgrass juice is considered the fountain of youth.

The molecules of chlorophyll found in wheatgrass juice and our own blood vary by just one element.

Chlorophyll has magnesium at the center, and our blood has iron at the center.

This is why wheatgrass juice helps you to recover from any illness. It just goes right into your bloodstream and begins to repair sick, diseased cells.

Things You Will Need— Where to Purchase Supplies.

Lowe's, Home Depot, Wal-Mart

- or home and garden store
- three-foot wire shelf with wheels (wheels may be extra)
- scissors or a very sharp knife for harvesting
- inexpensive potting soil or top soil (no need to purchase organic soil as it may contain mold)
- planting trays with drainage holes (Sometimes these big box stores will give you their leftover trays without cost to you, or you can go to a specialized seed store near you, or you can go online to Amazon.com and look up wheatgrass trays.)

- Approximate size would be 11"x 24"x 2" plastic with holes for drainage

Where to Buy Seeds and Kits
- www.gotsprouts.com
- www.wheatgrasskits.com
- organic, red, hard, winter wheat berry seeds are what many people use for wheatgrass
- organic, black oil, sun flower seeds are most recommended for the sunflower spouts

Special wheatgrass juicer
- Omega Juicer 8006, around $330.
- Google it for the best price.
- Other brands of wheatgrass juicers are available.
- Hand crank model by Lexen available for around $50 on the Internet

Some juicers can actually do fruits, vegetables, and wheatgrass. However, juicers specifically made for wheatgrass juicing give better results in the form of more juice and nutrients.

You will also need tightly woven stainless steel mesh colanders from any good kitchen supply store or a discount store. When you rinse the seeds, they won't fall through the holes as they would in regular pasta colanders.

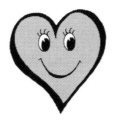

Appendix B

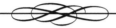

Suggested Reading

There is a wealth of information to be read on the subject of alternative health and spirituality. There are also many recipe books; some based on raw food preparation and some a combination of raw and cooked foods. The Internet is a huge resource for raw recipes. Use them all to find what you need.

I've read all the titles that are listed here and this is the information that came into my awareness when I needed it most. Your own research may include these among others. Pay attention to how you feel when deciding which books will be most beneficial on your own journey to improving your health. That *feeling* is one that causes you stop and take a second look and resonates in your heart. Happy reading and researching!

Health Related

Balch, Phyllis A., C.N.C. 2000. *Prescription for Nutritional Healing: A Practical A-to-Z Reference To Drug-Free Remedies Using Vitamins, Minerals, Herbs & Food Supplements.* New York: Avery.

Blaylock, Russell L. M.D. 2003. *Natural Strategies for Cancer Patients.* New York: Twin Streams Health.

Brantley, Timothy Dr. 2007. *The Cure: Heal Your Body, Save Your Life*. New Jersey: Wiley.

Clark, Hulda Regehr, Ph.D., N.D. 1993. *The Cure for All Cancers: Including Over 100 Case Histories of Persons Cured*. California: New Century Press.

Clark, Hulda Regehr Ph.D., N.D. 1995. *The Cure for All Diseases*. California: New Century Press

Dyer, David S. Dr. 2000. *Cellfood: Vital Cellular Nutrition for the New Millennium*. USA: Feedback Books.

Frahm, David and Anne Frahm. 1998. *Healthy Habits: 20 Simple Ways To Improve Your Health*. New York: Tarcher/Putnam.

Frahm, David and Anne Frahm. 1998. *Reclaim Your Health: Nutritional Strategies for Conquering Ailments*. New York: Tarcher/Putnam.

Gittleman, Ann Louise M.S., C.N.S. 2001. *Guess What Came To Dinner?: Parasites And Your Health*. New York: Avery.

Gittleman, Ann Louise Ph.D., C.N.S. 2000. *The Living Beauty Detox Program: The Revolutionary Diet for Each and Every Season of a Woman's Life*. New York: Harper San Francisco.

Griffin, G. Edward. 2006. *World Without Cancer: The Story of Vitamin B17*. California: American Media.

Henderson, Bill. 2008. *Cancer-Free: Your Guide to Gentle, Non-Toxic Healing*. USA: Booklocker.com.

Lee, John R. M.D. with Virginia Hopkins. 2004. *What Your Doctor May Not Tell You About Menopause: The Breakthrough Book on Natural Hormone Balance*. New York: Warner Wellness.

Lee, John R. M.D., David Zava PhD., and Virginia Hopkins. 2002. *What Your Doctor May Not Tell You About Breast Cancer: How Hormone Balance Can Help Save Your Life*. New York: Warner Books.

Lepore, Donald N.D. 1985. *The Ultimate Healing System: The Illustrated Guide To Muscle Testing & Nutrition.* Woodland Publishing, Inc.

Matwyshen, Joy. 2012. *Organic Gardening Made Easy.* Florida: Joy Matwyshen.

Quillin, Patrick PhD., R.D. and Noreen Quillin. 1994. *Beating Cancer With Nutrition.* Oklahoma: Nutrition Times Press.

Shinya, Hiromi M.D. 2010. *The Enzyme Factor: How To Live Long And Never Be Sick.* Canada: Council Oak Books.

Sumner, Jean. 2012. *52 Tips To Be Healthy.* South Carolina: Createaspace.com.

Sumner, Jean. 2013. *Journey To Raw: 52 Weekly Changes to add more raw food to your diet.* South Carolina: smashwords.com.

Voell, John R. 2003. *Cancer: How to Heal It, How to Prevent It.* Florida: Change Your World Press.

Voell, John R. and Cynthia A. Chatfield. 2005. *Cancer Report: The Latest Research, How Thousands are Achieving Permanent Recoveries.* Florida: Change Your World Press.

Wayne, Michael. PhD., L.Ac. 2005. *Quantum Integral Medicine: Towards a New Science of Healing and Human Potential.* New York: iThink Books.

Weil, Andrew M.D. 1997. *8 Weeks to Optimum Health: A Proven Program for Taking Full Advantage of Your Body's Natural Healing Power.* New York: Knopf.

Weil, Andrew M.D. 2001. *Eating Well for Optimum Health: The Essential Guide To Bringing Health And Pleasure Back To Eating.* New York: Quill.

Weil, Andrew M,D. 1995. *Spontaneous Healing: How to Discover and Enhance Your Body's Natural Ability to Maintain and Heal Itself.* New York: Fawcett Columbine.

White, Linda B. M.D. and Steven Foster and staff of Herbs for Health. 2000. *The Herbal Drugstore: The Best Natural Alternatives to Over-the-Counter and Prescription Medicines!.* USA: Rodale.

Willner, Robert E. M.D., Ph.D. 1994. *The Cancer Solution*. Florida: Peltic.

Winawer, Sidney J. M.D. and Moshe Shike, MD. 1995. *Cancer Free: The Comprehensive Cancer Prevention Program*. New York: Fireside.

Wolfe, David. 2009. *Superfoods: The Food And Medicine Of The Future*. California: North Atlantic Books.

Aromatherapy

Smith, Ed. 2009. *Therapeutic Herb Manual: A Guide to the Safe and Effective Use of Liquid Herbal Extracts*. Oregon: Ed Smith.

Worwood, Susan and Valerie Ann Worwood. 2003. *Essential Aromatherapy: a pocket guide to essential oils & aromatherapy*. California: New World Library.

Worwood, Valeria Ann. 1991. *The Complete Book of Essential Oils & Aromatherapy: Over 600 Natural, Non-toxic & Fragrant Recipes to Create Health, Beauty, A Safe Home Environment*. California: New World Library.

Spiritual References

Andrews, Andy. 2002. *The Traveler's Gift: Seven Decisions That Determine Personal Success*. Tennessee: Thomas Nelson.

Brown, Sylvia with Lindsay Harrison. 2004. *Prophecy: What the Future Holds for You*. New York: Dutton.

Burch, Wanda Easter. 2003. *She Who Dreams: A Journey into Healing through Dreamwork*. California: New World Library.

Byrne, Rhonda. 2010. *The Power*. New York: Atria.

Cota-Robles, Patricia Diane. 2010. *Who Am I? Why Am I Here?*. Arizona: eraofpeace.org.

Dyer, Wayne W. Dr. 2007. *Change Your Thoughts, Change Your Life: Living the Wisdom of the Tao*. California: Hay House.

Ford, Arielle. 2009. *The Soulmate Secret: Manifest the Love of Your Life with the Law of Attraction.* New York: Harper One.

Freeman, James Dillet. 2007. *The Story of Unity.* Missouri: Unity House.

Gaines, Edwene. 2005. *The Four Spiritual Laws of Prosperity: A Simple Guide to Unlimited Abundance.* USA: Rodale.

Giesemann, Suzanne. 2011. *Messages of Hope: The Metaphysical Memoir of a Most Unexpected Medium.* USA: One Mind Books.

Hartmann, Thom. 1999. *The Last Hours of Ancient Sunlight.* Great Britain: Hodder and Stoughton.

Hawkins, David R. M.D., Ph.D. 2002. *Power vs. Force: The Hidden Determinants of Human Behavior.* California: Hay House.

Hay, Louise L. 1999. *You Can Heal Your Life.* California: Hay House.

Hicks, Esther and Jerry Hicks. 2007. *The Astonishing Power of Emotions: Let Your Feelings Be Your Guide.* California: Hay House.

Hicks, Esther and Jerry Hicks. 2006. *The Amazing Power of Deliberate Intent: Living the Art of Allowing.* California: Hay House.

Hicks, Esther and Jerry Hicks. 2009. *The Vortex: Where the Law of Attraction Assembles All Cooperative Relationships.* California: Hay House.

Johnson, Timothy Dr. *2004. Finding God in the Questions: A Personal Journey.* Illinois: InterVarsity Press.

Katie, Byron with Stephen Mitchell. 2002. *Loving What Is: Four questions that can change your life.* New York: Three Rivers Press.

Khalsa, Dharma Singh M.D. and Cameron Stauth. 2001. *Meditation As Medicine: Activate the Power of Your Natural Healing Force.* New York: Pocket Books.

Lipton, Bruce H. Ph.D. 2008. *The Biology of Belief: Unleashing the Power of Consciousness, Matter & Miracles.* California: Hay House.

McCourt, Lisa. 2012. *Juicy Joy: 7 Simple Steps to Your Glorious Gutsy Self.* California: Hay House.

Murray, Maureen. 2004. *You Are Never Alone: Prayers and Meditations to Sustain You Through Breast Cancer.* Pennsylvania: Oncology Nursing Society.

Myss, Caroline Ph.D. 1996. *Anatomy of the Spirit: The Seven Stages of Power and Healing.* New York: Three Rivers Press.

Nohavec, Janet with Suzanne Giesemann. 2011. *Through The Darkness: My Tumultuous Journey from Roman Catholic Nun to Psychic Medium.* California: Aventine Press.

Nohavec, Janet with Suzanne Giesemann. 2010. *Where Two Worlds Meet: How to Develop Evidential Mediumship.* California: Aventine Press.

Osho. 2007. *The Buddha Said....:meeting the challenge of life's difficulties.* Great Britain: Watkins Publishing.

Perlmutter, Leonard with Jenness Cortez Perlmutter. 2005. *The Heart and Science of Yoga: A Blueprint for Peace, Happiness and Freedom from Fear.* New York: AMI.

Perron, Mari and Dan Odegard. *2001. A Course of Love.* California: New World Library.

Redfield, James. 1993. *The Celestine Prophecy: An Adventure.* New York: Warner.

Redfield, James. 1996. *The Tenth Insight: Holding the Vision.* New York: Grand Central Publishing.

Renard, Gary R. 2004. *The Disappearance of the Universe: Straight Talk about Illusions, Past Lives, Religion, Sex, Politics, and the Miracles of Forgiveness.* California: Hay House.

Renard, Gary R. 2006. *Your Immortal Reality: How to Break the Cycle of Birth and Death.* California: Hay House.

Tolle, Eckhart. 2005. *A New Earth: Awakening to Your Life's Purpose.* New York: Plume.

Tolle, Eckhart. 1999. *Practicing The Power of Now: Essential Teachings, Meditations, and Exercises from The Power of Now.* California: New World Library.

Tolle, Eckhart. 1999. *The Power of Now: A Guide to Spiritual Enlightenment.* California: New World Library.

Walsch, Neale Donald. 2005. *The Complete Conversations with God: an uncommon dialogue.* Virginia: Hampton Roads.

Wapnick, Kenneth Ph.D. 2004. *Ending Our Resistance To Love: The Practice of A Course in Miracles.* California: Foundation for A Course in Miracles.

Wapnick, Kenneth Ph.D. 2006. *The Arch of Forgiveness: The Practice of A Course in Miracles.* California: Foundation for A Course in Miracles.

Raw and Other Recipe Books

Alt, Carol. 2004. *Eating In The Raw: A Beginner's Guide To Getting Slimmer, Feeling Healthier, And Looking Younger The Raw-Food Way.* New York: Potter.

Baird, Lori and Julie Rodwell. 2005. *The Complete Book of Raw Food: Healthy, Delicious Vegetarian Cuisine Made With Living Foods—Includes over 350 Recipes From The World's Top Raw Food Chefs.* New York: Healthy Living Foods.

Brotman, Juliano with Erika Lenkert. 1999. *Raw: The UNcook Book: New Vegetarian Food For Life.* New York: HarperCollins.

Chavez, Gabrielle. 2005. *The Raw Food Gourmet: Going Raw for Total Well-Being.* California: North Atlantic Books.

Cohen, Alissa. 2006. *Living on Live Food.* Maine: Cohen Publishing.

Cornbleet, Jennifer. 2005. *Raw Food Made Easy: for 1 or 2 People.* Tennessee: Book Publishing.

Hyman, Mark MD. 2007. *The Ultra-Metabolism Cookbook: 200 Delicious Recipes for Automatic Weight Loss.* New York: Scribner.

Hyman, Mark MD. 2006. *Ultra-Metabolism: The Simple Plan for Automatic Weight Loss.* New York: Atria.

Malkmus, George with Peter and Stowe Shockey. 2006. *The Hallelujah Diet Workbook: Experience the Optimal Health You Were Meant to Have.* Pennsylvania: Destiny Image

McKeith, Gillian Dr. 2005. *You Are What You Eat: The Plan That Will Change Your Life.* New York: Plume.

Meyerowitz, Steve. 2007. *Sprouts: The Miracle Food The Complete Guide to Sprouting.* Massachusetts: Sproutman Publications.

Nungesser, Charles and Coralanne Nungesser and George Nungesser. 2005. *How We All Went Raw: Raw Food Recipe Book.* USA: In the Beginning Health Ministry.

Parragon. 2010. *Salads: A Collection of over 100 Essential Recipes.* Great Britain: Parragon.

Phyo, Ani. 2007. *Ani's Raw: food kitchen.* New York: Marlowe & Company.

Virtue, Doreen and Jenny Ross. 2009. *The Art of Raw Living Food: Heal Yourself and the Planet with Eco-delicious Cuisine.* California: Hay House.

APPENDIX C

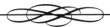

Websites for Alternative Services and Information and Recipes

The following websites are some of my favorites and those I first turn to when I have questions, but I explore others as well. Internet resources are plentiful and more than can be listed here. Again, do your own research and pay attention to how you feel when you're reading through them.

Services and Programs

www.annwigmore.org

www.cfnmedicine.com

www.drdach.com

www.gerson.org

www.hacres.com

www.HealthQuarters.org

www.hippocratesinst.org

www.sanoviv.com

Information

www.ajcn.nutrition.org

www.anh-usa.org

www.beautifulonraw.com

www.bioneers.org

www.cancure.org

www.chefelyse.com

www.counterthink.com

www.drdavidwilliams.com

www.drday.com

www.drhyman.com

www.energytimes.com

www.foodinvestigations.com

www.foodmatters.tv

www.fuelforthebody.org

www.gordonresearch.com

www.healthalert.com

www.healthforce.com

www.healthy-eating-politics.com

www.homegrownalmonds.com

www.hungryforchange.tv

www.justeatraw.com

www.lettucelove.us

www.loveatthecenter.com

www.johnleemd.com

www.mercola.com

www.nationalhealthfreedom.org

www.naturalnews.com

www.naturalnews.tv

www.naturalsociety.com

www.nutsonline.com

www.pcrm.org/health/diets/pplate/power-plate

www.rawguru.com/rawfoodrecipes.html

www.rawmazing.com

www.rawreform.com

www.RestoreOrganicLaw.org

www.rockinwellness.com

www.sickpills.com

www.surviveandthrivetv.com

www.theearthdiet.org

www.thenhf.com

www.therawfoodworld.com

www.therealfoodchannel.com

www.thrivemovement.com

www.totalhealthmethods.com

www.tropicaltraditions.com

www.vitacost.com

www.wake-up.tv

www.wayne-pickering.com

www.wilsonsthyroidsyndrome.com

www.worldwellnesseducation.biz

Documentaries on Alternative Health Information.

There are many more; the following are a few that I found most interesting and easiest to understand. (Most can be found, full-featured, on YouTube)

The Forbidden Cures

Cancer is Curable Now

Burzynski: Cancer is Serious Business FDA Tyranny

Food Matters

Food Inc.

Raw for 30 Days

Raw for Life

The Corporation

Eating

Healing Music

Frederic Delarue

"Musical Rapture, A Healing Gift to Humanity"
(Free download from Internet site.)

Plus several other CD's of music Frederic composed that can be purchased from www.fredericdelarue.com

Love At The Center

Free twelve minute meditation download with evidential medium Suzanne Giesemann and Frederick Delarue.

Plus other books and information related to letting go of fear and replacing it with unconditional love.

www.loveatthecenter.com or www.suzannegiesemann.com

Patchouli

www.patchouli.net
www.terraguitarra.com

Healing Artwork

Bruce Hecksel
www.terraguitarra.com/art

ABOUT THE AUTHOR

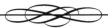

Linda Christina Beauregard

LINDA CHRISTINA BEAUREGARD GREW UP in the historic town of Bennington, Vermont located in the glorious Green Mountains. She spent most of her adult life as a wife and mother in Albany, New York while working as a legal administrator for a lobbying firm in downtown Albany for twenty-one years. She left that career to follow another passion, travel, and opened her own travel agency which she still operates.

Linda currently lives in sunny southwest Florida where her passion for dancing keeps her busy with ballroom, Latin and swing motions. As a Pisces, she frequents the beach and enjoys being surrounded by the dolphins and pelicans, salt water swimming, and all water related activities. Broadway musicals, art festivals, writing, traveling, and volunteering at local community theatre sustain her. She attends functions and services at Unity of Naples where the energy of unconditional love is so ever present.

As a breast cancer survivor she did the unthinkable. She went outside the norm of traditional surgery, radiation, chemotherapy, and other drug therapy to embark upon a journey that changed her life. She hopes her story will encourage and inspire you to investigate alternative options before making your final choice of treatments in the event you or someone you know is diagnosed with a life-threatening disease of any kind, not just cancer.

It's Linda's passion to share her journey so you can avoid harsh, chemical, traditional medical treatments and learn about the power of your own body. When given the right tools, you can create an absolute and complete healing. She wants you to be aware that you have other choices that mainstream medicine may not offer.

Linda is a Hallelujah Acres Health Minister and she started and ran a raw food club called Eating in the Raw with over 500 members. She enjoys speaking and teaching the importance of eating a plant based diet, avoiding a toxic lifestyle and how you can fend off and overcome disease using alternatives.

Linda has been a guest speaker at many women's and health clubs, and was a guest lecturer for Princess Cruises. Her story has appeared in newspaper articles, journals, on television and radio.

Linda will travel anywhere to share her story of recovery and encourage people to think and look outside the box for their healthcare needs. She can be reached at lindarawfood@gmail.com or on Facebook at Linda Christina Beauregard.

WORKS CITED

Abraham-Hicks. 2013. Accessed March 9, 2013.
http://www.abraham-hicks.com/lawofattractionsource/index.php

Blaylock, Russell L. Dr. 1997. *Excitotoxins: The Taste That Kills*. New Mexico: Health Press.

Blaylock, Russell L. Dr. "Excitotoxins: The Taste That Kills". YouTube video, 1:06:42. Posted July 10, 2011 by chronicalwatch.com. Accessed March 8, 2013.
http://www.youtube.com/watch?v=tTSvlGniHok

Borio Chiropractic Health Center. 2013. "Dairy – Milk, is "Udder" Nonsense". Accessed March 8, 2013.
http://www.boriochiropractic.com/Library/dairy.html

Braden, Gregg. 2008. Introduction to *The Spontaneous Healing of Belief: Shattering the Paradigm of False Limits*, xvii. USA: Hay House.

Braden, Gregg, "Gregg Braden-Quantum Healing of Tumour Thru the Power of Thought & Feeling". YouTube video, 9:31. Posted November 7, 2010 by Inspiritwellness. Accessed March 10, 2013.
http://www.youtube.com/watch?v=PZpRP1FV0lE

Brasscheck TV. 2009. "The sickest nation on earth?" *Americans for Constitutional Government Reform,* August 19, 2009, Accessed March 8, 2013.
http://a4cgr.wordpress.com/2009/08/20/07-106

breastcancer.org. 2013. Accessed March 8, 2013.
http://www.breastcancer.org

breastcancer.org. 2013. "IDC – Invasive Ductal Carcinoma". Accessed March 8, 2013.
http://www.breastcancer.org/symptoms/types/idc

Byrne, Rhonda. 2006. *The Secret.* New York: Atria.

Campbell, T. Colin PhD. and Thomas M. Campbell II. 2005. Introduction to *The China Study: Startling Implications for Diet, Weight Loss and Long-term Health,* 6. Texas: Benbella.

Cellulite Investigation. 2011. *"Healing Acne from Within—How to Diagnose and Cure Acne Caused by Fluoride Exposure".* Melissa. Cellulite Investigation. Accessed March 8, 2013.
http://www.celluliteinvestigation.com/wp-content/uploads/2011/11/A-Guide-to-Fluoroderma.pdf

Chopra Center Newsletter. 2011. "7 Secrets to Grow Younger, Live Longer". Deepak Chopra. Accessed March 9, 2013.
http://www.chopra.com/files/newsletter/May11/Newsletter-May11-deepak.html

Creative Methods. 2013. "US Air Quality Gradebook". Accessed March 8, 2013.
http://www.creativemethods.com/airquality/maps/index.htm

Dach, Jeffrey MD. 2013. "Wheatgrass" Jeffrey Dach MD. Accessed March 8, 2013.
http://www.drdach.com/Wheatgrass_8WDU.html

Day, Lorraine MD. 2013. Accessed March 8, 2013.
http://www.drday.com

Delarue, Frederic. 2009. *Eyes of Your Heart: Create a New Life Through the Eyes of Your Heart.* California: Frederic Delarue Productions.

Depaula, Suely, "Ho'o pono pono-Feel it!". YouTube video, 8:11. posted February 2, 2010, Accessed March 9, 2013.
http://www.youtube.com/watch?v=7Qoq75-DQm4&feature=related

drrossdc.com. 2013. "Mammograms and Breast Cancer". Dr. Calvin Ross. Accessed March 7, 2013.
http://www.drrossdc.com/Mammograms.htm

eHow.com. 2013. "What Is Fleece Fabric Made From?". Accessed March 8, 2013.
http://www.ehow.com/about_5080112_fleece-fabric-made.html

eHow.com. 2013. "What Is Multilevel Marketing". Heidi Wiesenfelder. Accessed March 8, 2013.
http://www.ehow.com/facts_5005885_what-multi-level-marketing.html

eHow.com. 2013. "What Is Polyester Fabric Made From?". Catie Watson. Accessed March 8, 2013.
http://www.ehow.com/facts_5792204_polyester-fabric-made-from_.html

ezHealthyDiet.com. 2007. "The Food Pyramid." T. Colin Campbell. Accessed March 7, 2013.
http://www.ezhealthydiet.com/food-pyramid.html

fluoridealert.org. 2012. "Brain". Accessed March 8, 2013.
http://www.fluoridealert.org/issues/health/brain

fluoridealert.org. 2012. "Fluoride & Intelligence: The 36 Studies". Michael
Connett and Tara Blank, PhD. Last modified December 9, 2012. Accessed
March 8, 2013.
http://www.fluoridealert.org/studies/brain01

fluoridealert.org. 2012. "Frequently Asked Questions". Accessed March 8, 2013.
http://www.fluoridealert.org/faq

Food & Thought. 2013. Accessed March 9, 2013.
http://foodandthought.com

Food & Thought, "Why Organic." *Vimeo* video, 5:04. Posted March 2011.
Accessed March 12, 2013.
http://foodandthought.com

Frahm, Anne E., and David J. Frahm. 1992. *A Cancer Battle Plan: Six
Strategies For Beating Cancer From a Recovered "Hopeless Case".*
Colorado: Pinon.

Frahm, Dave. 2000. "Air and Water Purification Strategies." In *A Cancer
Battle Plan Sourcebook: A Step-By-Step Health Program To Give Your
Body A Fighting Chance,* 161-166. New York: Tarcher/Penguin.

Frahm, Dave ND, MH, CNC, CNHP. 2009. *The Breast Cancer Pattern: It
Starts With Your Starving Thyroid.* Colorado: HealthQuarters Ministries.

Frederic Delarue. 2012. "Private Spiritual Tours of the Desert". Accessed
March 10, 2013.
http://www.fredericdelarue.com

Gerson Institute. 2013. Accessed March 8, 2013.
http://gerson.org/gerpress

Giesemann, Suzanne. 2013. "The Ten-Minute Transformation". Accessed March 9, 2013.
http://www.suzannegiesemann.com/meditation.html

Gittleman, Ann Louise, and Smith, Melissa Diane. 1999. *Why Am I Always So Tired?: Discover How Correcting Your Body's Copper Imbalance Can... *Keep your body from giving out before your mind does *Free you from those midday slumps *Give you the energy breakthrough you've been looking for.* New York: HarperCollins.

Graham, Douglas N. Dr. 2006. *The 80/10/10 Diet: Balancing Your Health, Your Weight, and Your Life, One Luscious Bite at a Time.* Key Largo: FoodnSport Press.

Gucciardi, Anthony. Is There Really a Difference Between Organic and Conventional Food?". YouTube video, 9:35. Posted September 4, 2012. Accessed March 10, 2013.
http://www.youtube.com/watch?v=8PmqUA8qfRQ

HealthQuarters Ministries. 2013. Accessed March 8, 2013.
https://www.healthquarters.org

Howell, Edward Dr. 1985. *Enzyme Nutrition: The Food Enzyme Concept.* USA: Avery.

Newhart, Bob, "Bob Newhart-Stop It!". YouTube video, 6:21. Posted September 1, 2010 by Josh Huynh. Accessed March 10, 2013.
http://www.youtube.com/watch?v=Ow0lr63y4Mw

Jensen, Bernard D.C., PhD. 1981. "Chapter 3, Autointoxication." In *Tissue Cleansing Through Bowel Management: With The Ultimate Tissue Cleansing System*, 20-23. Tennessee: Healthy Living Publications.

Jensen, Bernard D.C., PhD. 1981. "Chapter 4, Constipation." In *Tissue Cleansing Through Bowel Management: With The Ultimate Tissue Cleansing System*, 26-37. Tennessee: Healthy Living Publications.

livestrong.com. 2013. "What Emotions Affect Different Organs In The Human Body?". Jeffrey Traister. Accessed March 9, 2013. http://www.livestrong.com/article/193234-what-emotions-affect-different-organs-in-the-human-body

livinglibations. 2012. Accessed March 8, 2013. http://www.livinglibations.com

Mercola.com. 2013. "Does Milk Really Look Good On You?". Ingri Cassel. Accessed March 10, 2013. http://articles.mercola.com/sites/articles/archive/2000/02/27/no-milk.aspx

Mercola.com. 2013. "Sunscreen & Tanning". Accessed March 8, 2013. http://shop.mercola.com/catalog/sunscreen-tanning,142,0.htm

Mercola.com. 2013. "Warning Never Swallow Regular Toothpaste". Accessed March 8, 2013. http://articles.mercola.com/sites/articles/archive/2009/04/07/warning-never-swallow-regular-toothpaste.aspx

Mercola.com. 2013. "Why did the Russians Ban an Appliance Found in 90% of American Homes?". Accessed March 10, 2013. http://articles.mercola.com/sites/articles/archive/2010/05/18/microwave-hazards.aspx

Mercola.com. 2013. "Why You Should Avoid Root Canals Like the Plague". Accessed March 8, 2013.
http://articles.mercola.com/sites/articles/archive/2010/11/16/why-you-should-avoid-root-canals-like-the-plague.aspx

Miller, Jim. "How to Grow Wheatgrass – Jim Miller". YouTube video, 30:01. Posted January 8, 2012 by WorldWellnessEd. Accessed March 8, 2013.
http://www.youtube.com/watch?v=R1ysca2lidI

National Geographic. 2013. "Chemicals within Us". David Ewing Duncan. Accessed March 8, 2013.
http://science.nationalgeographic.com/science/health-and-human-body/human-body/chemicals-within-us.html

Natural News.com. 2013. "Baby boomers - Why detoxifying toxins from your early years could save your life". Ethan A. Huff. Accessed March 7, 2013.
http://www.naturalnews.com/037047_detoxification_baby_boomers_cleansing.html

Natural News.com. 2013. "Celebrity-branded perfumes loaded with toxic petrochemicals". David Gutierrez. Accessed March 8, 2013.
http://www.naturalnews.com/030635_perfumes_toxic_chemicals.html#ixzz20ATLEhGz

Natural News.com. 2013. "Higher US drug spending has not improved health". Jonathan Benson. Accessed March 8, 2013.
http://www.naturalnews.com/030324_drug_spending_health.html

Natural News.com. 2013. "Prescription drug deaths skyrocket 68 percent as Americans swallow more pills". M.T. Whitney. Accessed March 8, 2013.
http://www.naturalnews.com/021635.html#ixzz1uaO5npPU

Natural News.com. 2013. "The racket that is Big Pharma". Sherry Baker. Accessed March 8, 2013. http://www.naturalnews.com/037373_Big_Pharma_racket_prescription_drugs.html

Natural News.com. 2013. "Twenty-seven years brings no deaths from vitamins but over three million from pharmaceuticals". Anthony Gucciardi. Accessed March 8, 2013. http://www.naturalnews.com/034372_vitamins_pharmaceuticals_deaths.html

Natural News.com. 2013. "Why and how microwave cooking causes cancer". Paul Fassa. Accessed March 8, 2013. http://www.naturalnews.com/030651_microwave_cooking_cancer.html

OpenSecrets.org. 2013. "Agribusiness". Accessed March 7, 2013. http://www.opensecrets.org/lobby/indus.php?id=A&year=a

OpenSecrets.org. 2013. "Agricultural Services/Products". Accessed March 7, 2013. http://www.opensecrets.org/lobby/indusclient.php?id=A07&year=2012

OpenSecrets.org. 2013. "Food Processing & Sales". Accessed March 7, 2013. http://www.opensecrets.org/lobby/indusclient.php?id=A09&year=2012

OpenSecrets.org. 2013. "Lobbying Database". Accessed March 7, 2013. http://www.opensecrets.org/lobby/index.php

Owens, Brandi. "The correct way to skin brush!" YouTube video, 11:28. Posted December 4, 2011 by GreenSmoothieGirl. Accessed March 8, 2013. http://www.youtube.com/watch?v=AZfMhXsjXeQ&feature=youtu.be

Patchouli. 2013. Accessed March 9, 2013.
http://www.patchouli.net

Patchouli. 2013. "Patchouli's Band Biography". Accessed March 9, 2013.
http://www.patchouli.net/bio

Ph In Balance. 2010. "What is Live Blood Analysis". Accessed March 8, 2013.
http://www.ph-inbalance.com/what-is-live-blood-analysis

Powers, Richard. 2010. Accessed March 8, 2013.
http://www.richardpowers.com

Real Food Channel. 2013. "The Best Diet". YouTube video, 9:01. Posted October
23, 2012 by The Real Food Channel. Accessed March 8, 2013.
http://www.therealfoodchannel.com/videos/the-science-of-healthy-eating/
the-best-diet.html

Rodale Institute. 2013. "The Farming Systems Trial: Celebrating 30 years".
Accessed March 9, 2013. http://rodaleinstitute.org/our-work/farming-
systems-trial/farming-systems-trial-30-year-report

Ruiz, Don Miguel. 1997. *The Four Agreements: A Toltec Wisdom Book.*
California: Amber-Allen.

Ruiz, Don Miguel, Don Jose Ruiz and Janet Mills. 2010. *The Fifth
Agreement: A Practical Guide to Self Mastery.* Amber-Allen: California.

Salt Cave. 2012. Accessed March 8, 2013
http://www.saltcave.us

Schucman, Helen. 1976. *A Course in Miracles.* California: Foundation for
Inner Peace.

Stanford Dance. 2010. "Use It or Lose It: Dancing Makes You Smarter". Richard Powers. Accessed March 2013. http://socialdance.stanford.edu/syllabi/smarter.htm

Suite101. 2013. "Xenoestrogens and Your Health". Linda Beadle. Accessed March 8, 2013. http://suite101.com/article/list-of-xenoestrogens—chemical-estrogens-a205523

SweetPoison.com. 2010. Accessed March 8, 2013. http://www.sweetpoison.com

Trudeau, Kevin. 2004. *Natural Cures "They" Don't Want You To Know About.* Illinois: Alliance.

truthinlabeling.org. 2013. "Names of ingredients that contain processed free glutamic acid (MSG)". Last modified February 2011. http://www.truthinlabeling.org/hiddensources.html

Wikipedia. 2013. "Margarine". Accessed March 10, 2013. http://en.wikipedia.org/wiki/Margarine

INDEX

Cancer iii, ix, xi, xii, xiii, xv, xvii, xviii, xxi, xxiii, xxiv, xxv, 3, 5, 7, 11, 12, 13, 14, 15, 16, 17, 18, 19, 21, 22, 23, 24, 25, 26, 27, 28, 30, 32, 33, 35, 38, 39, 40, 41, 42, 44, 45, 46, 47, 49, 50, 58, 59, 61, 64, 79, 81, 92, 93, 95, 96, 97, 98, 106, 115, 119, 122, 127, 133, 136, 141, 142, 143, 144, 145, 146, 152, 156, 157, 159, 161, 162, 164, 173, 188, 189, 190, 193, 194, 199, 200, 203, 204, 205, 206, 207, 208, 211, 212, 213, 214, 215, 216, 217, 229, 230, 231, 232, 234, 239, 241, 242, 245, 246, 250

Cancer Battle Plan 27, 59, 211, 246

Candida 40, 120, 123, 126

Candle 97, 156

Canned 50, 51, 52, 57, 84, 96, 164, 165, 175

Carageenan 52, 53

Carbohydrate xv, 47, 79, 117, 122, 165, 175, 206

Carboxyl 90

Carcinogen 49, 58, 59

Carcinogenic 91

Carnivore 39

Cascara sagrada bark 125

Catalyst 163, 164, 182

Cat scan 17

Caustic 96, 97, 146

Cell xvi, 13, 15, 17, 18, 19, 24, 30, 36, 37, 46, 47, 51, 52, 53, 65, 67, 78, 79, 94, 95, 96, 108, 110, 125, 135, 136, 139, 143, 145, 149, 155, 156,

162, 163, 164, 165, 166, 172, 182, 184, 188, 200, 203, 216, 227

Challenge xii, xxiv, 72, 112, 131, 136, 158, 186, 234

Chamomile flower 125

Characteristic 139

Chemical xx, xxi, xxii, xxiv, xxv, 28, 30, 41, 47, 49, 50, 55, 59, 60, 61, 64, 65, 66, 74, 76, 82, 84, 85, 86, 87, 88, 89, 90, 91, 103, 104, 105, 109, 112, 123, 125, 147, 163, 164, 167, 168, 170, 172, 173, 177, 178, 179, 182, 183, 195, 201, 209, 210, 216, 242, 249, 252

Chemistry 88, 149, 160

Chemotherapy xii, xiii, xvii, xxv, 7, 15, 23, 26, 27, 31, 33, 95, 96, 97, 142, 193, 200, 241

Chest X-ray 17, 24

Chew 66, 176, 193, 205

Chicken 39, 53, 57, 63, 126, 127, 178, 207

China Study xxii, 58, 178, 244

Chinese 58, 110, 149, 216

Chlorine 59, 109, 123, 176, 177, 225

Chlorophyll 94, 95, 227

Cholesterol 11, 40, 48, 93, 100, 101, 102, 113, 120, 121, 122, 217

Cholesterol deposits 40, 100, 101, 102, 113, 122

Chopra, Deepak 162, 208, 216, 244

Chronic 65, 72, 127, 163, 167, 209

Circumstance 35, 37, 70, 71, 123, 131, 143, 147, 149, 153, 155, 187, 190, 194

Cleaning product 47, 65, 85

117, 125, 126, 128, 166, 167, 173, 175, 179, 181, 182, 184, 201, 207, 209, 216, 219, 229, 230, 231, 232, 233, 249, 250, 252

Natural bristle brush 110

Natural fiber 91

Natural flavor 51, 54

Natural spice 50, 51

Natural sugar 117, 175

Naturopath 29, 30, 35, 44, 126, 145, 216

Naturopathic Doctor 29, 35, 126, 145, 216

Nausea 102

Negative 48, 50, 52, 72, 99, 135, 136, 137, 138, 140, 142, 148, 149, 150, 153, 154, 161, 177, 188

Newhart, Bob 186, 247

Nipple 19, 32

non-Hodgkin 95, 203, 212

Noninvasive 21, 29, 145

Nontoxic 79, 82

Note to My Soul 201, 202

Nucleus 94, 136

Nuisance 136

Nut 43, 68, 121, 125, 167, 193, 210

Nutrient xviii, 21, 45, 48, 51, 57, 77, 79, 84, 95, 96, 117, 118, 119, 127, 135, 164, 165, 166, 173, 175, 176, 179, 180, 184, 205, 219, 228

Nutritional 44, 47, 51, 71, 73, 95, 103, 105, 161, 172, 179, 207, 226, 229, 230

Nutritionist 27, 35, 42, 43, 44, 219

O

Obesity 33, 57, 58, 118

Ohm 152

Oil 28, 66, 68, 69, 75, 86, 87, 88, 90, 91, 97, 101, 109, 112, 123, 139, 175, 181, 182, 184, 190, 228, 232

Old age 42, 43, 44

Olive 66, 68, 88, 101, 184

Oncologist 12, 14, 15, 16, 17, 18, 31, 32, 144, 145, 203, 211, 215, 216

Opportunity xi, xviii, 107, 158

Optimum 64, 97, 176, 231

Organic xi, xii, xiii, xviii, xxii, xxiv, xxv, 21, 37, 39, 43, 45, 51, 52, 53, 69, 71, 74, 79, 80, 82, 87, 88, 98, 101, 103, 104, 105, 116, 123, 127, 128, 129, 143, 146, 149, 165, 168, 169, 170, 171, 172, 173, 174, 176, 178, 179, 181, 184, 190, 191, 207, 209, 210, 227, 228, 231, 246, 247

Organically grown xxi, xxii, 59, 63, 126, 172, 173, 179, 191

Organism 102, 126, 136

Orthopedic 26

Osteoporosis xiii, 3, 48, 50, 73, 77, 188, 219, 220

Outdated 141

Overload xxiii, 97, 106

Oxidize 95

Oxygen 60, 67, 78, 79, 94, 95, 108, 110, 135, 177, 206, 214

Oxygenate 78, 153

P

Packaging 88, 89, 182

Pancreas 90, 165

Para Cleanse 120, 125

Paradigm 159, 187, 243

Paralyze 41

Parasite 37, 113, 119, 120, 123, 124, 125, 126, 127, 230

Passion xi, 40, 104, 107, 129, 155, 156, 193, 210, 214, 241, 242

Pasteurize 179, 180, 181

Pasture animals 127

Patchouli 160, 240, 251

Pathology 18, 19, 24

Pattern xix, 20, 30, 44, 45, 46, 71, 137, 190, 246

Paw paw 125

Peace 36, 38, 97, 137, 142, 147, 153, 158, 159, 169, 202, 205, 234, 251

Peak efficiency 25, 47, 98, 99, 101, 102, 124, 184

Pensive 150

Perception 136

Perfume 47, 88, 249

Period 16, 17, 49, 73, 194, 209

Peroxide 123

Personal care 47, 88, 91

Pessimistic 50, 140

Pesticide xx, xxi, 47, 59, 91, 123, 127, 170, 172, 178, 179

Petroleum 89, 90, 97, 112

pH 44, 48, 58, 73, 74, 131, 156, 230, 232, 233, 234, 235, 251

Pharmaceutical xxiii, xxiv, xxv, 27, 30, 38, 50, 56, 59, 64, 71, 103, 250

Pharmacy 50, 101

Philosophies 151, 218

Phlebitis 16

Phosphoric acid 48

Phosphorous 73, 180

Phthalates 88

Physical iv, xii, 14, 24, 33, 36, 37, 40, 47, 93, 102, 106, 107, 135, 137, 140, 141, 150, 155, 156, 173, 185

Physical activity 106

Plant xii, 2, 25, 58, 59, 60, 66, 117, 123, 125, 126, 163, 168, 173, 174, 200, 201, 217, 224, 226, 242

Plastic 47, 61, 89, 90, 94, 96, 97, 99, 114, 121, 183, 223, 226, 228

Plastic surgery 61, 183

Poison 18, 24, 61, 67, 85, 86, 103, 112, 132, 170, 172, 178, 201, 204

Poison control center 61, 85, 112

Political 38, 151

Politics 138, 234, 238

Pollute xxiii, 167

Pollution xxi, 95, 167

Polyester 90, 245

Polymer 90

Pores 66, 69, 84, 86, 89, 90, 109, 110

Positive 15, 16, 40, 100, 125, 126, 130, 137, 140, 143, 149, 161, 177, 188, 193, 196, 197, 201

Power xii, xiv, xxii, 2, 25, 39, 80, 107, 108, 126, 133, 151, 156, 187, 190, 193, 194, 196, 197, 200, 201, 217, 231, 232, 233, 234, 235, 238, 242, 243, 251, 252

Powerful xii, xvii, xxv, 21, 39, 58, 59, 68, 96, 117, 130, 132, 143, 144,

X

Xanthine oxidase 180
Xenoestrogen 90, 91, 252
X-ray 6, 9, 14, 17, 21, 22, 24, 136, 191,
    192

Y

Yeast 40

Z

Zinc 44, 45, 47, 219